AF477171

PHARMACOGNOSY
LAB MANUAL

PHARMACOGNOSY
LAB MANUAL

M.A. IYENGAR & S.G.K. NAYAK

Department of Pharmacognosy
College of Pharmaceutical Sciences
Manipal - 576 119.

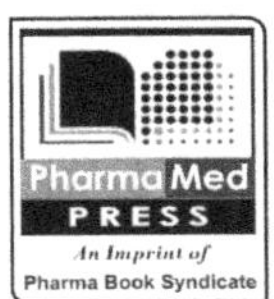

PharmaMed Press

An imprint of Pharma Book Syndicate

A unit of BSP Books Pvt. Ltd.
4-4-309/316, Giriraj Lane,
Sultan Bazar, Hyderabad - 500 095.

Published by

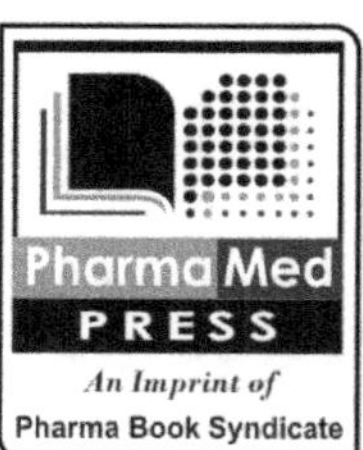

PharmaMed Press

An imprint of Pharma Book Syndicate

A unit of BSP Books Pvt. Ltd.
4-4-309/316, Giriraj Lane, Sultan Bazar, Hyderabad - 500 095.
Phone: 040-23445600/688; Fax: 91+40-23445611
E-mail: info@pharmamedpress.com
www.pharmamedpress.com/pharmamedpress.net

ISBN: 978-93-86819-53-6 (Hardbound)

PREFACE

In our constant endeavours to systematize the study of Pharmacognosy, we feel, this is one more innovative approach. It is customary that before the practical class begins, the concerned teacher gives instructions as to what all should be done for a particular drug. The instructions are usually written on a black board and the students come and spend considerable time in copying. A big class means several batches and all that to be repeated with a manual like this, the student knows before entering the practical class his assignments which he should carry out systematically without anyone's help, provided he is motivated.

Students should get a meaningful and at the same time joyful learning experience of finding out things for themselves. So we teachers have to adopt suitable methodology to stimulate the students both in our lecture - and practical classes. This approach we are sure, will bring-in the desired competence in the student. The attention of the student is drawn to various significant differences, peculiar exceptions and precautionary measures to be observed. Further, in some of the institutions, the study of Pharmacognosy is covered according to the Laboratory facilities and convenience. Sometimes the students remain ignorant of the necessary information, it is not then the students fault that they are ignorant of some facts, some information and some technique. This will serve as *a* reminder *as* to what is expected of one. Needless to mention here that this manual is an accompanying book to the other popular books authored by us. For the first time we are giving here the technical details of the TLC studies followed by us here for years now. A rich experience of over two decades has gone into this book, the first of its kind in the country. When taken in the right spirits, we are sure, this book would serve by and large the student community and also the teaching fraternity.

While this manual has been done in a very short time, just to meet the demands and needs of the present batch of students, a press printed version of the same is on its way.

With immense pleasure, we place on record our heartfelt thanks to Mr. Pattabhi Rama Rao M. Pharm., for the excellent Computer Print-outs and the work connected with that. It is only because of him, we could expedite this publication. Our sincere thanks are also to Mr. Dayanand Pai, Chief Librarian; Staff, Computing Centre, KMC, Manipal and M/s. Prasad Photostat, Udupi for their kind help and ready service.

- Authors

CONTENTS

Quantitative Microscopy

GENERAL INSTRUCTIONS

I. Requirements:

For the laboratory work you are required to equip with the following materials:

1. Practical Record Book (200 pages – 27 cm × 22 cm).
2. Practical observation note book.
3. Writing materials (pen, pencil, eraser, color pencils, scale etc.).
4. A clean Napkin (a piece of white cloth 1/2 metre).
5. A clean Apron.
6. A sharp blade/scalpel, a camel-hair brush, dissection needle, match box etc.
7. Books – Study of Crude Drugs (SCD)

    Anatomy of Crude Drugs (ACD)
    Pharmacognosy of Powdered Crude Drugs (PCD)
    Pharmacognosy Lab Manual (PLM)

II. Lab Discipline:

1. For practical work see that you are equipped with the above mentioned lab materials.
2. For successful performance, come fully prepared for the day's work.
3. Submit completed records of the previous week's work to the perusal of your teacher.
4. Spread the napkin on the working table and keep china dish, watch glass, slides, coverslips, brush, needle etc. on it.
5. Listen to the instructions properly or copy the instructions in the observation book.
6. Handle the microscope, TLC plates, Jars, Spray-bulbs, micrometers, Camera Lucida, UV lamp etc. with extra care.
7. It is possible at times while cutting sections, you may injure one of your fingers. See that there is always medicated plaster in your pencil box for ready use.
8. Do not keep the reagent bottles at the working spot. After use bring them back to their original places.
9. Handle the inflammable solvents with extra care. Do not bring them near the flame.

10. Work systematically, try to understand all aspects of the practical work scheduled for a particular day/drug and clarify your doubts then and there only. This is the main advantage of the contact hours. Do not hesitate to take help from your teachers.

11. It is said Cleanliness is next to Godliness. Keep your working table neat and clean. With that 50% success is achieved. Throw unwanted materials, wastes in the dust bin kept in your vicinity.

12. Complete the day's assignment within the given period and do not carry forward anything for the next day.

13. Unless there is a specific reason/unavoidable reason, do not absent yourself for practical, as it is difficult to repeat the same practicals again.

14. Be in your seats 10 min. earlier than the scheduled time so that you settle well before you begin.

WHAT ALL YOU SHOULD KNOW ABOUT THE MICROSCOPE YOU WOULD BE USING EVERYDAY?

The most important instrument constantly used in a pharmacognosy lab is the compound microscope. Assuming that the students are quite familiar with the parts and functioning of this optical instrument, it's diagram and description is avoided. However, some of the important tips to handle this expensive instrument are given here.

1. Being a sensitive instrument, you have to handle it carefully.

2. Keep the microscope in a proper place where artificial or natural light is available to focus it.

3. Rotate the nose-piece and bring the low power objective (shorter one, 10 X) to the middle of the stage resting 1 cm above the stage level.

4. Move the substage condenser up, keep the iris diaphragm fully open and looking through eye piece (10 X) focus with the help of concave mirror till the entire field of view is uniformly illuminated.

5. Take a clean glass slide with the material mounted in the centre, and place it horizontally on the central portion of the stage, just below the objective or above the condenser.

6. While observing through the eye piece, keep both the eyes open so as to avoid strain on one eye.

7. Looking through the eye piece move the draw tube upwards using the coarse adjustment knob, till a clear picture of the material appears. Adjust the illumination/cut down the light by lowering the condenser down or by closing the aperture of the iris diaphragm partially or by adjusting the concave mirror. Do not keep the objective higher up and move it downwards. You are likely to break the coverslip and spoil the material and objective tip. Do not observe any material without putting a coverslip.

8. Check up whether the material mounted is in the proper perspective (i.e., not in the inverted position).

9. Look into your specimens especially sections properly and see whether it is complete of incomplete, transversely cut or obliquely cut, free from air bubbles or not etc.

10. Keep your ACD next to your microscope and study all the tissues one by one systematically.

11. Some characters such as Cal. oxalate crystals, pollen grains, starch grains, aleurone grains, exact nature of stomata etc. which may not be

normally seen under LP, are then to be observed under high power objective (HP, longer objective- 40X).

12. To observe under· HP, slowly rotate the nose piece and bring the objective to the middle of the stage. This objective being longer than the LP objective, almost touches the coverslip. Therefore you have to use only fine adjustment knob for fine focussing of the tissues. See that the upper surface of the coverslip is clean otherwise the CH or stain will spoil the HP objective tip.

13. After use, immediately rotate the nose piece and bring back the LP objective. Never leave the microscope anytime under HP objective.

14. After completing your work, see that the slides are removed from the stage and return a clean microscope.

SYSTEMATIC APPROACH TO STUDY THE PRACTICAL ASPECTS OF DRUG IN THE LAB

Organized Drugs

(a) **Source, constituents and uses:** Study the source i.e., the part of the plant, the botanical name and family: brief knowledge of the constituents and uses as given in SCD.

(b) **Morphology:** Observe the morphological characters taking good specimens (fresh, dried or museum specimens) of the drug and draw diagrams as given in SCD and describe them.

(c) **Transverse Sections:** Method of taking transverse sections is given for certain drugs wherever necessary (for eg; leaves, barks etc.). Also refer 'The General Account for Leaves' on page 9.

Mounting Technique: Thin sections are placed on the glass slide, few drops of chloral hydrate soln. is added and warmed over a micro burner and gently boiled until it clears. Add more chloral hydrate soln. if it evaporates during the process. Place a coverslip carefully on the material avoiding air bubbles.

Absorb excess reagent with a piece of blotting paper otherwise chloral hydrate recrystallizes when it dries up. The mountant/reagent should not be there on the coverglass or underside of the slide.

For staining, add 2-3 drops of Phloroglucinol to the cleared section and then add 2-3 drops of con. HCl and put back the coverslip. One could also prepare first a 1:1 mixture of Phloroglucinol and Con. HCl and use it. Final mount is always either in CH soln. or Glycerin. Extra care is to be taken to see that all the excess of this staining mixture out side the cover slip is removed with the help of a blotting paper. Otherwise the con. HCl will spoil the stage and objectives of the microscope. All lignified tissues take up red color but then the calcium oxalate crystals dissolve and disappear. To observe starch grains, mount the sections in water, put the coverslip, add a drop of Iodine soln. to one edge of the coverslip and blot out the solution from the other side of the coverslip. Starch present take up blue color. The above said preparations are likely to dry up after sometime. To avoid this a thin film of Glycerin may be made around the coverslip on its outer edges by which the specimens may be preserved for few hours.

As said above, prepare 3 slides (i.e., CH, Stained and one for starch where present) for every drug. Study the tissues as given in ACD. Report to your concerned teacher your performance and results. Please show the sections in their proper perspectives and not in a slanting or inverted Positions.

(d) Powder: Mount a very small amount of powder and prepare 2 to 3 slides in CH soln., Phloroglucinol + HCl and Iodine water (if necessary) as per the procedure mentioned above. Refer PCD and study all the identification characters. Call your teacher, who will always be at your service, and clarify your doubts.

(e) Chemical Tests: Perform the chemical tests/microchemical tests wherever required or mentioned either individually or in groups and report and record your observations.

(f) Thin layer chromatographic techniques (General Introduction):

TLC is a very commonly used chromatographic technique for the analysis of mixture, separation of mixtures and identification of individual constituents. The method is extremely rapid and visual evaluation is very easy. Why is this method so popular? Reasons are many:

(i) Time required is very short.

(ii) One can roughly estimate the quantity of an individual constituent present.

(iii) One can detect easily the purity of a drug. It is easy to separate out the adulterant from the authentic drug by TLC technique.

(iv) One can preserve the results for a long time.

(v) Cost wise, it is very cheap. No major equipments required. Simple in operation, less time consuming, very sensitive too and finally it requires minimum laboratory space.

The principle involved in TLC is same as that of Paper Chromatography. The only difference is the supporting media is inorganic here and that has added advantage. Usually separations can be achieved with a solvent run of 10 cm. which may require one hour. Some of the commonly used adsorbents are Silica gel, Kieselguhr, Alumina, Cellulose and Polyamide. A suitable slurry is made with the adsorbent and this slurry is spread evenly on a glass plate. Of course, some equipments are available to control the uniformity of the layer. And abroad, ready machine made plates are also available, the price of which would be exhorbitant in India. What we normally use in our lab is silicalgel G which includes approximately 13% Calcium sulfate as binding agent. The prepared plates are air dried for sometime and then are to be activated by heating them at 110 $^{\circ}$C for atleast 1 h. The activated plates must be kept over a desiccant in a closed cabinet.

Application: Trim the plate by holding the plate in one hand and wiping out the extra silicagel layer on the sides with a finger. Solutions of extracts and reference standards are applied by means of fine capillary tube, taking care not to disturb the layer. Better apply several times at the same spot rather than applying once a big spot. On a single application, the spot has to be dried by blowing a gentle stream of air. To economize, we ask two students to put their plates back in one jar. Replace the lid as fast as possible so as not to disturb the saturated atmosphere. What should be depth of solvent in the jar? Although this is not the students problem, but they should know the theory behind this. The depth should be such that the solvent surface is about 1 cm below the spots on the plate. After the desired run of 10 cm or so, remove the plate from the jar, note the solvent front before it gets dried and allow it to dry finally. It is customary to observe the spots, if any, under UV before spraying. Spray the plate now with a suitable detection reagent and observe the color pattern. One more advantage of inorganic supporting media is the use of corrosive spraying reagents without any problem. This cannot be done with a paper chromatogram.

Find out the Rf value of the compounds in question by comparing with authentic compounds. Rate of flow is the distance moved by the solute divided by distance moved by solvent front of a compound, determined under specific conditions. This being reasonably specific from 0.1 to 0.99

Practical Instructions:

TLC plates are to be handled carefully. Do not use the bottom portion of silica gel to write any indication marks. This disturbs the flow of the solvent. The details can be written on the upper most portion of the silica gel using a pointer. Apply the extracts and test substances/standard solutions spacing out properly above 1.5 to 2 cm. from the bottom of the plate (the bands or the spots of extracts applied should not be dipped in the solvent mixture). Avoid applying on the extreme left or right sides. The developing jars should normally contain 30 to 40 ml of the solvent mixture which is already saturated. One jar is to be shared by two students. Keep the jars on your working table in such a place where it remains undisturbed throughout the development time. Take care that the jar is not kept next to a Bunsen burner. Keep both the plates back to back inside the jar simultaneously. Replace the lid immediately, as otherwise the saturated atmosphere changes. Keep a cheek on the run of the plate. Normally the plates develop in 30-45 min. (except Ephedra where it takes 2 h.). The solvent must flow atleast upto 10 cm from the point of application.

Once the plates are developed, remove both the plates simultaneously and replace the lid of the jar. Dry them in air for 15-20 min. and if required in an oven. Cool before spraying. While spraying the plate, the sprayer bulbs are to be handled carefully. Spray the plate thoroughly and properly inside a fuming cupboard. Take extra care while spraying corrosive reagents like H_2SO_4, HNO_3 etc.

Whenever plates are to be heated, place them in an oven carefully without disturbing other plates kept by others. When proper colors appear, take out the plate with the help of a forceps, tongs or napkin. Proper colors are of importance particularly when we are dealing with essential oils. Wherever UV lamp is used, handle it carefully. If you are required to note the spots under UV lamp, take a pointer and mark the entire spot with dots all around. Show the plates to your concerned teacher, take Rf values and record them. Reproduce the plate with proper colors in your record book immediately.

Unorganized Drugs:

General instructions are given under appropriate chapter. Show all the tests to your concerned teachers and get them evaluated. Record the tests and results in a tabular column as given in the manual.

Miscellaneous Drugs:

Write the source, constituents and uses of the drugs given in your syllabus with the help of SCD. Observe Their morphological characters.

Quantitative Microscopy:

Detailed instructions are given at the appropriate place.

Record Writing:

Organized Drugs:

Always write the description part on the ruled page (pen) and diagrams on the blank page (pencil). Always at the top of the page, write the name of the drug and below that subtitles like morphology, TS, Powder and TLC etc. should appear. Further, on the left corner at the top of each fresh page the botanical name of the drug will come and then on the right hand corner, the family to which it belongs.

For each drug write on the 1st page:

Morphological sketches. For this refer SCD. Draw diagrams to the natural size if they are big enough. In case of small specimens (like Isapgol, Santonica) in order to show the characters properly diagrams can be magnified and the magnification has to be mentioned at the bottom of the diagram (for eg. Santonica inflorescence × 10). Space out the diagrams properly. Captions for each diagram are to be written at its bottom and underlined. Label the different parts of the diagrams. Draw straight lines to label the parts. Do not use zig zag lines and intersect them. No pen to be used on this page.

On the 2nd page draw a neat labelled diagram of the TS of the drug as shown in ACD. Write the description on ruled page.

Utilize the 3rd page for the powder characteristics. Here also the page should have the title and subtitle. For powder characters refer PCD. Description on the ruled page.

Fourth and final page is for TLC experiment. Keep the size of the chart uniform throughout (15 cm × 6 cm). Draw the point of application, solvent front, size of spots, appropriate colors and Rf values. Refer PLM (Pharmacognosy Lab Manual).

Unorganized Drugs:

Source, morphology, constituents, uses on the ruled page. On the unruled page write the title, physical tests and chemical tests (in tabular form).

Miscellaneous Drugs:

They are to be covered in the last few pages of the record (Count the required number of pages for organized drugs, unorganized drugs and miscellaneous drugs and use the record accordingly). For miscellaneous drugs, write only the source, constituents and uses both on ruled and unruled pages.

LEAF DRUGS

General Account

I. Morphology:

(a) Type of leaf - simple, compound, pinnately compound, palmately compound.

(b) Condition - fresh/dried.

(c) Shape - ovate, lanceolate , cordate etc.

(d) Petiole - petiolate /sessile.

(e) Margin - entire, dentate, wavy etc.

(f) Apex - acute, acuminate, mucronate etc.

(g) Base - lamina base equal, unequal etc.

(h) Surface - upper (ventral) – color, nature, glabrous etc.

lower (dorsal) - color, nature, glabrous etc.

(i) Venation - reticulate-pinnate, palmate, parallel etc.

(j) Size - length, breadth.

(k) Odor

(l) Taste

(m) Any other special characters-dotted glands, marginal veins etc.

Draw diagrams to their natural size.

II. Surface preparation:

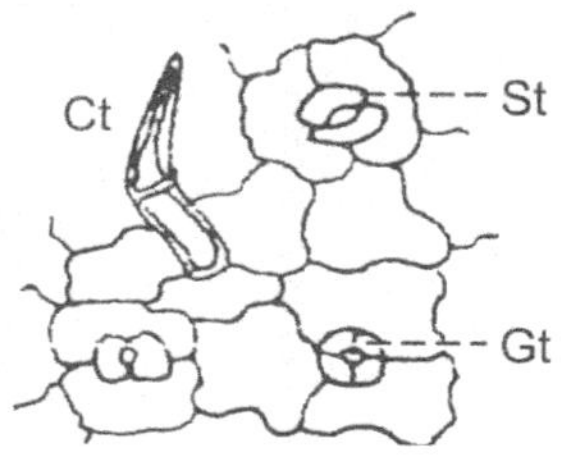

A peeling of the lower epidermis is to be mounted in chloral hydrate (CH) soln. Observe and record the type of stomata, covering and glandular trichome if any (draw few stomata long with the surrounding epidermal cells and trichomes if any).

III. Microscopy:

To study the anatomical details of a leaf, one has to take a thin transverse section passing through midrib along with a portion of lamina on either side. A slab of potato/the mocol may be used as a pith to support the leaf pieces so that sections can be taken easily. Split two third portion of potato piece as shown in the figure and insert the leaf piece in such a manner that the cut surface is horizontal. Hold the potato piece with the leaf piece inside, in your left hand between the thumb and index finger. Hold the sharp blade between the right hand thumb and index· finger. Cut thin and complete sections horizontally all along the lamina and midrib, along with the potato piece. Keep both blade and material wet by frequently dipping in water. Transfer the sections from the blade to watch glass containing water. Check the potato piece after cutting few sections. If you have been getting oblique sections, once again cut the potato slab horizontally and continue cutting the sections. In this way take 20 to 30 sections within 10-15 min.

Pick up 3 to 4 sections on a glass slide, add CH saln. boil thoroughly for few minutes. Plenty of air bubbles appear, if not cleared properly. When CH evaporates, add more CH. Place the section in the middle of the slide (parallel to the slide in case of leaf sections) and put the coverslip slowly with the help of a needle avoiding the appearance of air bubbles. Remove excess of CH with a blotting paper and observe under a microscope (LP objective). Retain one good section. Transfer other good sections carefully to another slide, add 2-3 drops of phloroglucinol followed by equal volume of Con. HCl. Set it aside for 3 to 5 min. The stained sections are now to be mounted either in CH or Glycerin. Put on a coverslip again carefully and observe under a microscope. Leaf sections being very delicate, extra care is to be taken while clearing, staining, putting coverslip etc.

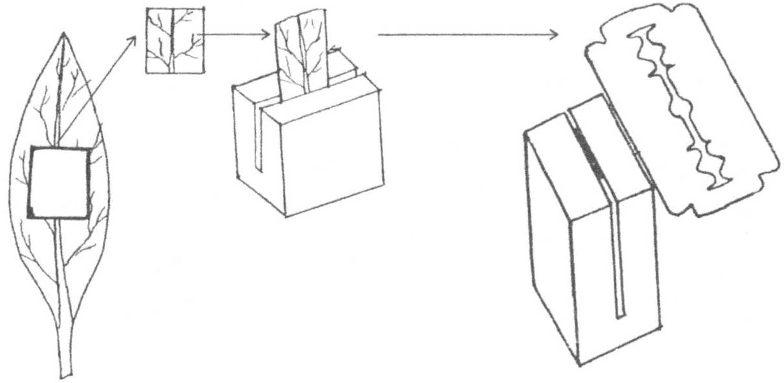

EPIDERMAL TISSUE SYSTEM

Epidermal tissue system consists of the outermost covering or skin of the various plant organs called as 'epidermis'. It is this layer which has the contact between the environment and plant body. Primarily this is a protective tissue. Except for the stomatal pores, the epidermis is a continuous layer, normally made up of a single layer of compactly arranged tabular of lenticular cells without any intercellular spaces.

I. **Epidermal Tissue System:**

   A: Type of Epidermal Cells:

   (i) Simple Epidermal Cells:

   eg. Datura. Mount the upper epidermal layer of the leaf.

   (ii) Beaded Epidermal Cells:

   eg. Digitalis lanata (Powder).

   The anticlinal walls of the epidermal cells have thickening giving the appearance of beads.

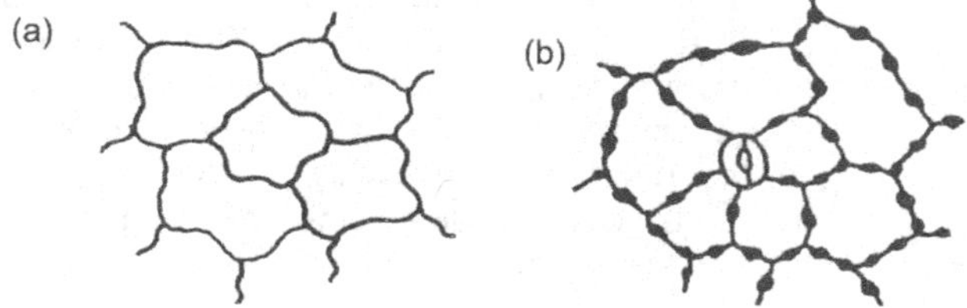

Fig. 1

   B: Study of Trichomes:

   Trichomes are plant hairs and are elongated epidermal outgrowths consisting of a portion embedded in the epidermis called as foot and a free projecting portion called the body. In the pharmacognostical study trichomes are of immense help in the identification of drugs as they are specific to certain drugs.

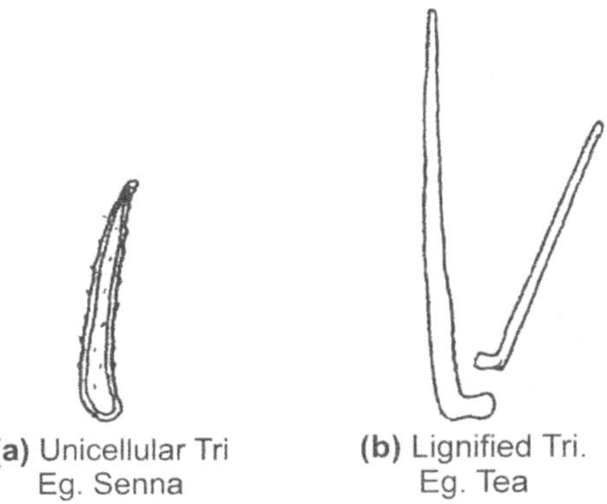

Fig. 2

Trichomes are of two types:

(i) The Covering trichomes:

These are usually protective in function and may be unicellular or multicellular.

(a) unicellular trichomes:

eg. Senna (powder or epidermal peeling).

(b) unicellular lignified trichomes: eg. Tea (powder).

(c) Multicellular trichomes:

eg. Datura (epidermal peeling).

(d) Branched trichomes:

eg. Verbascum (powder). These consist of central uniseriate axis from which side branches arise. Also called as Candelabra trichomes.

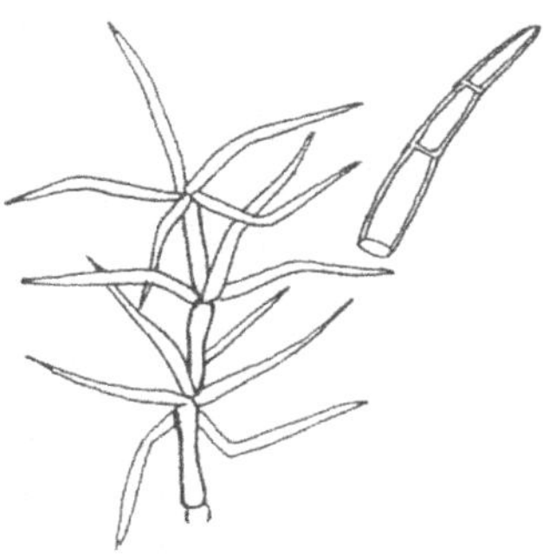

Fig. 3

(e) Collapsed trichomes: Certain cells of the trichomes are collapsed or have become placid. eg. Digitalalis purpurea (powder).

(ii) Glandular Trichomes:

These are secretory in function.

(a) Sessile: Glandular trichomes are small, sessile with quadricellular heads.

eg. vasaka (epidermal peeling)

(b) Multicellular and uniseriate: eg. Digitalis purpurea (powder) and Datura (epidermal peeling).

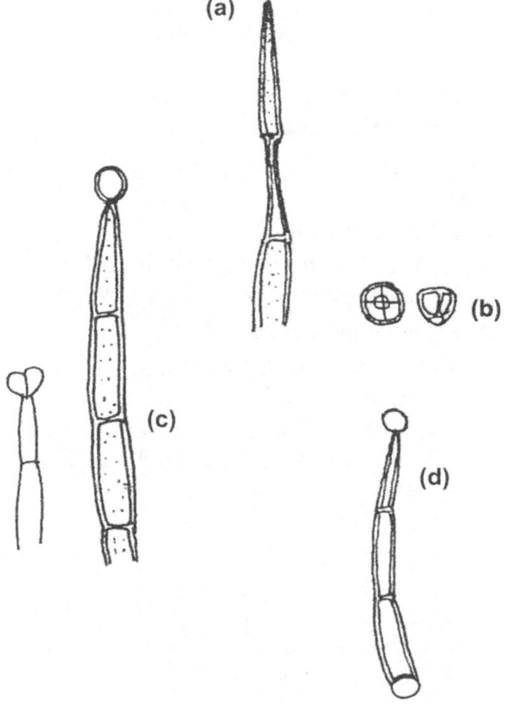

Fig. 4

C. Stomata:

Stomata are openings in the epidermal layer. As these are also specific to particular plants, these act as diagnostic characters, in the identification of drugs. Each stoma (sing.) is made of a pair of guard cells enclosing a small pore called as stomal pore. The epidermal cells surrounding the stoma are called subsidiary cells. Depending upon the number and arrangement of subsidiary cells in relation to stoma, there are 4 types of stomata:

(i) Anomocytic (Ranunculaceous) or Irregular Celled Type:

Here the stoma is surrounded by more than three subsidiary cells which are irregularly arranged and cannot be differentiated from other epidermal cells.eg. Eucalyptus (epidermal peeling).

(ii) Anisocytic / Cruciferous / Unequal Celled Type:

This type of stoma consists of 3 subsidiary cells of which one is smaller than the other two. eg. Datura (lower epidermal peeling).

(iii) Paracytic / Rubiaceous / Parallel - Celled Type:

The stoma here has two subsidiary cells, the long axis of which lie parallel to the guard cells . eg. Senna (epidermal peeling).

(iv) Diacytic / Caryophyllaceous/Cross- Celled Type:

Here again two subsidiary cells at right angles to the axis of stoma. eg. Vasaka (lower epidermal peeling).

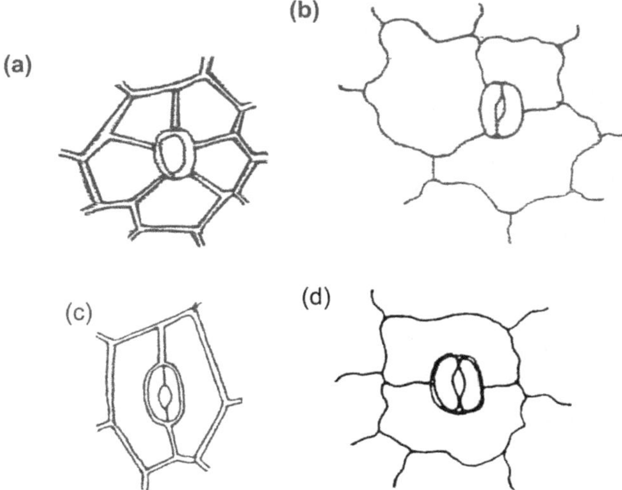

Fig. 5

II. Ergastic Substances:

These are non protoplasmic cell contents and being specific to certain drugs, are of immense help in the identification.

(i) Cystolith: It is the aggregation of calcium carbonate crystals. eg.Vasaka (clearly seen in the longitudinal section and TS of the petiole mounted in water). Both in HCl and $CH_3 COOH$, it dissolves giving effervescence.

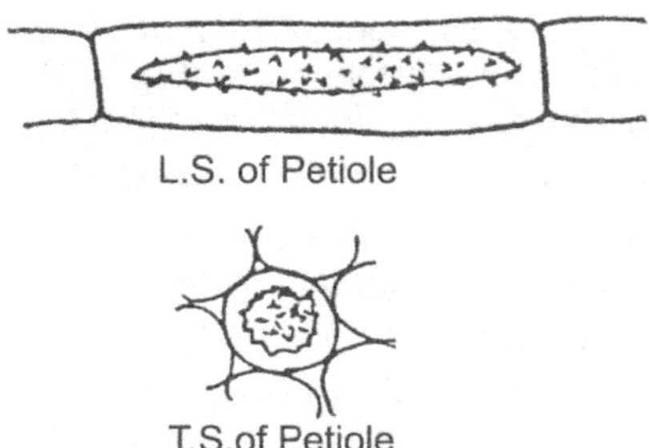

Fig. 6

(ii) Calcium oxalate crystals: Occur in dirrerent forms. Unlike calcium carbonate these are soluble in HCl with no effervescence and insoluble in $CH_3 COOH$.

(a) Prisms: Calcium oxalate crystals in the form of prisms.eg: Quillaia and Senna (powders).

(b) Cluster crystals: These are aggregates of numerous prisms in the form of a spherical mass which have projecting points and angles.
eg: Senna (powder), Datura (TS).

(c) Acicular raphides: calcium oxalate crystals in the form of needles. eg: Squill (powder)

(d) Microsphenoidal crystals: These are small solitary crystals occurring in a cell in large numbers, sometimes completely fill the cells.
eg: Sandy balls of Belladonna (powder).

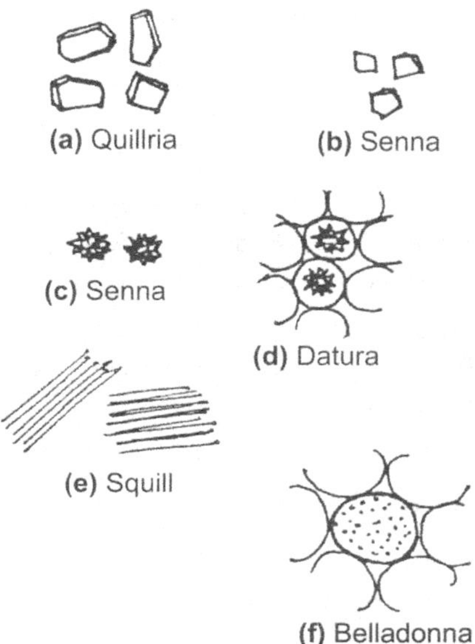

Fig. 7

DIGITALIS

Digitalis purpurea   Fam: **Scrophulariaceae**

1. Morphology :   Observe fresh (if available) or dried (herbarium) leaf. Salient features given in SCD are to be observed and recorded in your journal.

2. Powder   :   Observe the color, odor and taste of the powder. Mount the powder in CH and study the identifying characters as indicated in PCD.

Record your observations and draw the same.

Record; Page I – 1; II – 2

Digitalis lanata

1. Morphology :   Here again observe fresh (if available) or dried specimens and note the salient features.

Draw an entire leaf in your journal.

2. Powder   :   Observe the color, odor and taste of the powder. As usual mount the powder in CH and study the identifying characters as indicated in PCD.

Record your observation and draw the same.

Record : Page I-1; II-2

Note: While ***D. purpurea*** powder can be identified on the basis of the typical collapsed trichomes, the adulterants like ***Verbascum thapsus*** and ***symphytum officinale*** show branched trichome called as candelabra in case **Verbascum** and unicellular hook shaped trichomes in ***Symphytum.*** These are to be noted if the adulterants are available. Powder of ***D. lanata*** can be identified based on beaded epidermal cells.

EUCALYPTUS

Eucalyptus species   Fam: **Myrtaceae**

1. Morphology   :   Observe salient external features of a fresh leaf as indicated in SCD. Draw a neat labelled diagram in your journal.

2. TS   :   Mount in chloral hydrate to observe prisms and cluster crystals. Mount in phloroglucinol + HCl (1:1) to observe the lignified tissues like; Xylem vessels and pericyclic fibres. Also note the disappearance of prisms and cluster crystals in the stained section. Study the different tissues as indicated in ACD and draw a neat labelled diagram in your record.

**3. Surface
   preparation**   :   It is difficult to take a peeling of the epidermal layers of the leaf. Therefore scrape the upper or lower epidermal layer with the help of a blade and mount the transparent piece of the leaf in chloral hydrate. Observe and draw the characteristic epidermal cells along with the anomocytic stomata (PCD character No.2)

4. Powder   :   Mount both in chloral hydrate and later in phloroglucinol and HCl. Study the identifying characters as indicated in PCD.

5. Distillation   :   Observe the distillation of the Eucalyptus oil from the fresh leaves and note the nature of the oil (Take 100g. of leaves and find out the % yield of the oil.)

6. TLC of the oil :   Adsorbent: Silica gel plate

Solvent system: Toluene (or Benzene) + Ethyl acetate (93 : 7). Take 30 ml (27.9 + 2.1) in the jar and saturate atleast for 1 h.

Application: Applied in the form of spots.

Eucalyptus oil (diluted in toluene or chloroform in the proportion of 1:10): 10 µl Cineole (1: 30 dilution in same solvent): 10 µl

Running distance: 10 cm.

Euc. oil   cineole

Cineole

$$\frac{a}{b} = \frac{7.8}{10.5}$$

$$= 0.742$$

Drying: Air drying for 15 min. and later in an oven for 3 to 5 minutes.

Detection: Cool the plate, spray thoroughly with vanillin H_2SO_4 and heat at 110 °C for 5-10 min. under observation till blue colored spots appear.

Caution: Whole plate turns violet if over heated.

Record Rf of Cineole (approx. 0.7) in visual light and draw the chromatographic chart in your record.

SPOT OUEST IONS ON TS:

Describe the TS of Eucalyptus.

On what basis would you identify the TS of Eucalyptus leaf ?

Which are the lignified tissues in the TS?

What is meant by isobilateral leaf?

What is the active constituent here and where exactly it is located?

Bring out the differences between a stained and an unstained section.

Why do you think this is a TS?

Why do you think this is TS of a leaf?

Name the ergastic substances in the TS.

Diagrams in the record:

Page – I - 1,3 ; II – 2; III – 4; IV – 5,6

MENTHA

Mentha species   Fam: **Labiatae**

For want of fresh specimen, both morphology and TS are usually not done in the practical class.

1. Powder : (A) Observe the color, odor and taste of the powder
(B) Mount the powder in CH and study the identifying characters as indicated in PCD. Record your observations and draw the same.

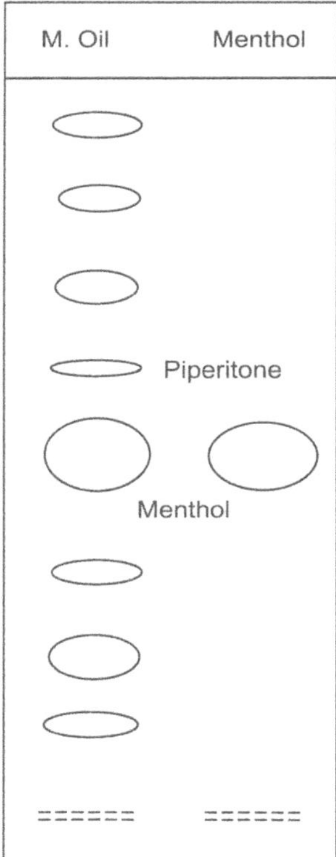

2. TLC of Mentha oil: Observe the color and odor of the oil.

Adsorbent: Silica gel plate.

Solvent system:

Toluene: Ethyl acetate (93: 7). Chromatographic jar to be saturated for 1 h.

Mentha oil to be diluted in the proportion of 1:10 in toluene or chloroform and 10 µl of this applied in band form.

Menthol, also diluted in 1:5 ratio in toluene or chloroform and 10 µl of this applied in band form.

Running distance: 10 - 12 cm.

Drying:

Air drying for 15 - 20 min. and then in oven for 3 to minutes.

Detection: Spray thoroughly with vanillin - H_2SO_4 reagent. Heat at 110 °C - for 5 to 10 min. under observation (do not over heat). Observe in visual light for blue colored spots of menthol and a small orange colored spot of piperitone just above menthol.

Record Rf value of menthol (approximately 0.4 - 0.5)

NOTE: Powder illustrations to be done on one page and TLC chart to be shown on a different page.

Record: Page I - 1; II - 2

SENNA

Cassia angustifolia   Fam: **Leguminosae**

1. Morphology : Observe the salient external features of a fresh leaflet (if available) or of a dry leaflet as indicated in SCD. Draw a neat labelled diagram in your record. Also observe the dried pods (fruits) which also contain the active constituents hence used in medicine.

2. TS: Dried leaflets are to be soaked for 20 to 30 min. in water and then sections are to be taken. The sections being very delicate are to be handled carefully while transferring to the glass slide, clearing, staining or while placing the cover - slip.

Observe in: CH preparation: Cluster crystals in mesophyll crystal sheath in the midrib

Stained preparation: Lignified tissues like xylem vessels, sclerenchyma in the midrib region and vascular strands in the lamina region.

Observe all the tissues and draw a neat labelled diagram in your record as given in ACD.

3. Surface
**   Preparation :** Observe and draw the characteristic epidermal cells along with paracytic stomata and unicellular trichomes.

4. Powder: Observe the color, odor and taste. Mount the powder in chloral hydrate and also in phloroglucinol + HCl. Study the identifying characters as indicated in PCD.

5. Chemical
**   Test :** Senna being an anthraquinone containing drug it is customary to perform the so called anthraquinone test or Borntrager's test (refer SCD). However, instead of powder as mentioned therein, one could also perform the test by taking the crushed leaflets.

6. TLC of Senna: **Preparation of the extract:**

0.5 g. of leaf powder is extracted by warming for 10 min. on water bath with 5 ml of methanol (50%). The filtrate is used for TLC.

Solvent system:

n - propanol: ethyl acetate: water (4:4:3)

Application: all in band form Senna extract: 20 µl

Sennoside A (1% dilution in MeOH): 10 µl

Sennoside B (1% dilution in MeOH): 10 µl (or mixture of sennoside A and B)

Running distance: 15 cm.

Drying: Air drying for 20 min In oven for 5 min.

Detection:

Cool and first spray with 25% HNO_3 and heat the plate for 10 min. at 120 °C (do not overheat). Cool the plate, again spray with 10% methanolic KOH solution and warm the plate carefully.

6 to 7 reddish brown and yellow spots are seen in visual light.

Record Rf values of

Sennoside A (approx. 0.4) and

Sennoside B (approx. 0.2)

Record: Page I - 1,3; II - 2; III - 4, 5 ; IV - 6

SOLANACEOUS DRUGS

Datura metel var. fastuosa   Fam: **Solanaceae**

1. Morphology :   Observe the general morphological features of the plant in general and then the salient features of the leaf in particular as given in SCD. Draw a neat labelled diagram in your record.

**2. Microscopy
   of the leaf** :   A thin TS to be mounted in CH solution and the different types   of   calcium   oxalate   crystals   -   prisms, microsphenoidal crystals (sandy balls) and cluster crystals are to be noted. There after the section is to be stained in the usual way and the lignified tissue, here namely the xylem vessels only, to be noted. Draw the TS as in ACD and label the parts.

**3. Surface
   preparation** :   This is done to see the epidermal cells in surface view and so also the individual trichomes both covering and glandular and the cruciferous (anisocytic) stomata. For this peeling of the leaf to be mounted in chloral hydrate. Record your observation in your journal.

Powder Study: The powders of the following drugs are always to be cleared thoroughly with strong chloral hydrate till the pieces of lamina are clear enough to show the type of calcium oxalate crystals,based on which the Solanaceous drugs can be identified.

**4. Datura
   stramonium** :   Observe cluster crystals in a particular pattern in the mesophyll region.

**5. Hyoscyamus
   niger** :   Observe prisms also in a particular pattern in the mesophyll region.

**6. Atropa
   belladonna** :   Observe sandy balls in the mesophyll. The market samples of dried Belladonna leaves usually contain the leaves of the adulterant - **Phytolacca decandra**. These however, can be identified on the basis of bundles of acicular raphides in the mesophyll region.

Use full page to draw these features as in PCD

7. TLC Studies of Solanaceous drugs :

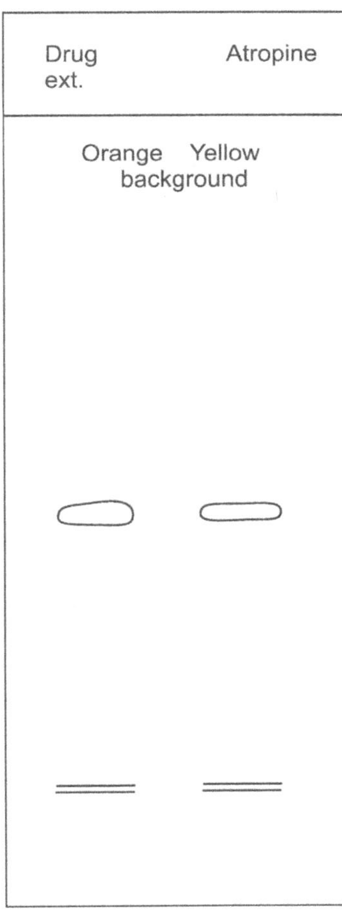

Preparation of extract:

Take 2 g. of powdered drug and shake for 5 min. with 10 ml of 0.05 NH_2SO_4 and filter. Add 1 ml concentrated ammonia solution to the filtrate. Dilute the mixture to 10 ml with water and extract by shaking with 10 ml ether. Dry the ethereal layer over Na_2SO_4 (anhydrous). Filter and evaporate the filtrate to dryness on a water bath. Dissolve the residue in 0.5 ml methanol.

Adsorbent: Silica gel plate.

Solvent system: Toluene: Ethyl

acetate: Diethylamine (7:2:1).

Application: To be applied in band form

Drug extract: 30 µl

Atropine standard (1% atropine sulphate in methanol): 10 µl

Running distance: 10 cm.

Drying: Air drying for 15-20 min. and then in oven for 3-5 min.

Detection: Cool the plate and first spray with Dragendorff's reagent; as the spots are unstable, plate is sprayed again with 1% Sodium nitrite solution.

Record Rf value of atropine in visual light. (Atropine takes brownish violet color. Approximate Rf value varies from 0.4 to 0.6 depending upon the saturation).

Diagrams in the journal:

Page I - 1, 3; II - 2; III - 4; IV - 5; V – 6

(draw mesophyll tissue of, Phytolacca showing acicular raphides); VI – 7.

SQUILL

Urginea indica   Fam: **Liliaceae**

1. Morphology : Observe the entire plant, both the fresh bulbs and dried slices of the bulb as described in SCD and draw neat labelled diagrams in your record.

2. Microscopy : TS of the fresh scale leaf to be taken and mounted.

(a) one in CH solution to observe the characteristic acicular raphides (needle shaped crystals)

(b) one in phloroglucinol + con. HCl so as to see the lignified xylem vessels.

(c) one in ruthenium red to observe the fact that inspite of a mucilaginous drug, this mucilage here does not take any color; however with corallin soda, the mucilage does take the red color.

(d) one in Iodine solution. The mucilage present in the parenchymatous mesophyll takes up reddish purple color while that present in European squill does not take any color. Thus this is a distinguishing test.

Draw a neat labelled diagram in your record using ACD as the model.

3. Powder : Observe the color, odor and taste and record these observations. Also look for bundles of acicular raphides in a chloral hydrate preparation, that being the characteristic feature of Squill. Draw this in your record (PCD).

Record: Page I - 1; II - 2; III – 3.

TEA

Camellia sinensis (Syn : Thea sinensis)   Fam: **Theaceae**

1. Powder   :

    a) Observe the color, odor and taste of the powder

    b) Mount the powder in CH and phloroglucinol + con. HCl and study the identifying characters as indicated in PCD. Record your observations and draw the same.

**2. Chemical
   test**   :

Normally this test is not done in the laboratory in view of the use of potassium chlorate. However one is expected to know this test - Murexide Test. An extract of tea or for that matter even coffee is taken on a small watch glass and to this few drops of HCl is added and there after one or two crystals of potassium chlorate. The watch glass is kept on a water bath in a fume cupboard so as to evaporate the contents of the watch glass to dryness. Caffeine, the ophylline and the obromine - purine alkaloids - give a purple color.

3. TLC of Tea / Coffee / Purine alkaloids:
Preparation of the extract: 2g.of the drug (tea/coffee) is taken in a flask containing 10 ml mixture of ethanol: chloroform: water (4: 2: 1) and heated on a water bath and filtered. The residue on the filter paper is washed with the same mixture, so as to make 15 ml of the filtrate. This filtrate is to be applied directly.

Adsorbent: Silica gel

Solvent system:

Ethyl acetate : Methanol : Water (100: 16.5 : 13.5). Take 39 ml in the proportion of (30: 5: 4). Chamber to be saturated for 1h.

Application : In band form.

Tea/Coffee extract - 20 µl

Caffeine (I% in MeOH/ CHCl$_3$): 10 µl

Running distance: 10 cm

Drying: Air drying for 20 min and later in an oven for 3 to 5 minutes and the plate to be cooled before spraying.

Detection : First spray with alcoholic iodine solution and alter 2 min. with alcoholic HCl. Record Rf values of caffeine (chocolate brown spots with approx. Rf value 0.7) in visual light. If the spots disappear after spraying with alcoholic HCl spray again with alcoholic iodine.

Record: Page I - 1; II - 3.

VASAKA

Adhatoda vasica   Fam: **Acanthaceae**

1. Morphology :

Observe salient external features of a fresh leaf as indicated in SCD. Draw a neat labelled diagram in your record.

2. TS :

Sections to be mounted in chloral hydrate, water (to see cystolith) and phloroglucinol and HCl. Also take a thin LS or TS of the petiole and mount in water specially to observe cystolith, the peculiar feature of Vasaka. Observe the different tissues as seen in the TS (ref. ACD) and draw a neat labelled diagram in your record.

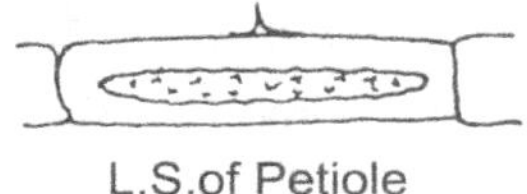

L.S.of Petiole

3. Surface
Preparation :

Mount the lower epidermal peeling in chloral hydrate solution, observe & draw type of stomata, epidermal cells, covering trichomes and glandular trichomes.

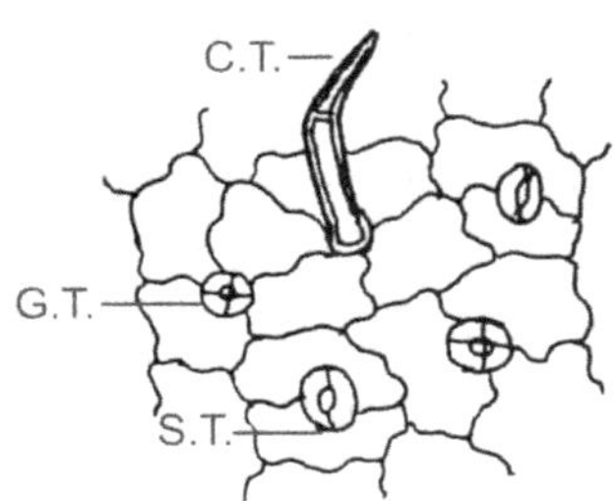

4. Powder :

Observe the color, odor and taste. Mount the powder in chloral hydrate and also in Phloroglucinol + HCl. Study the identifying characters as indicated in PCD.

5. TLC :

Preparation of the extract: Take 5 g of the powdered leaf and basify with ammonia. After drying, extract with 20 ml of chloroform: isopropanol (3:1) in warm condition. Filter the extract, concentrate the filtrate and use for TLC studies.

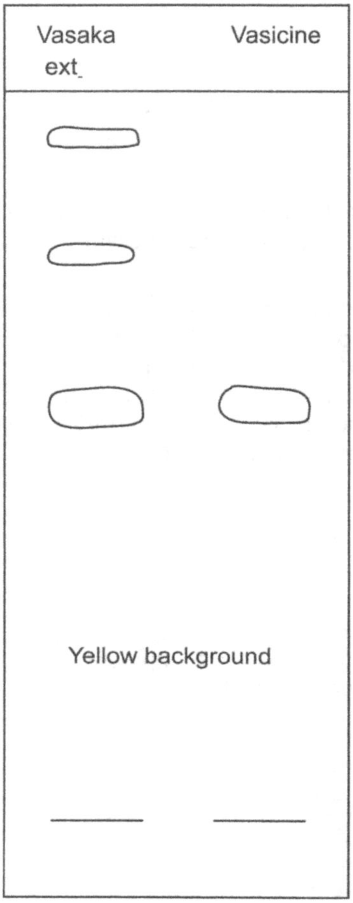

Vasaka ext.	Vasicine

Yellow background

Adsorbent: Silica gel pate.

Solvent System:

(a) Toluene/benzene: Ethyl acetate: Diethylamine (7:2:1) or

(b) Dichloromethane: methanol (3:1) Take 30 ml in a chamber and saturate for atleast an hour.

Application: To be applied in band form

Vasaka extract - 20 μl

Vasicine (1% CH_3OH soln.) - 10 μl

Running distance: 10 to 12 cm.

Drying: Plates are air dried for 15 min and then in an oven for 5 min.

Detection: Cool the plate and spray with Dragendorff 's reagent or keep the plate in Iodine chamber.

Observation:

(a) With Dragendorff's reagent 3 prominent orange brown colored spots appear in the Rf range between 0.4 and 0.95

(b) Treatment with iodine vapour also shows 3-4 spots in the same Rf range.

Record:

The Rf value of Vasicine (approx. Rf value is between 0.45 and 0.7 depending upon the solvent system and saturation of the chamber).

Reproduce the plate in the journal with yellow background and orange colored spots.

Record: Page I - 1,3 ; II - 2 ; III - 4 ; IV - 5

FLOWER DRUGS

CLOVE

Eugenia caryophyllata   Fam: **Myrtaceae**

1. Morphology : Observe

    (a) an entire flower bud

    (b) L.S. of a bud

        (observe with hand lens) - Ref.SCD.

    (c) Mother clove

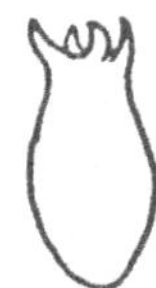

    (d) Clove stalk

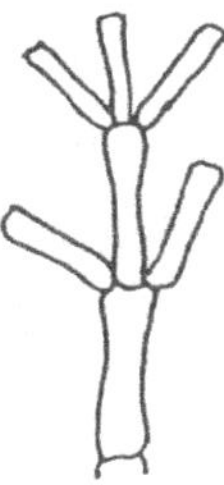

2. Microscopy : Flower buds soaked overnight are to be used for taking TS.

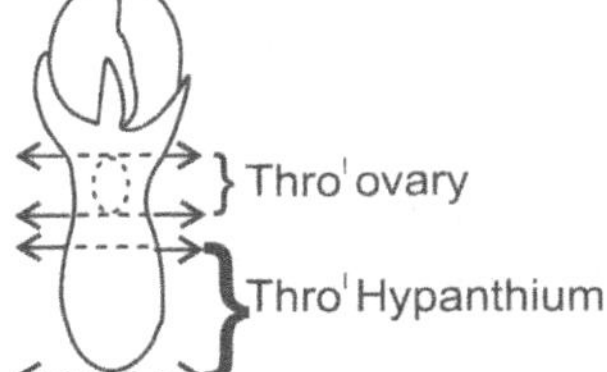

Take a TS passing through hypanthium and one another section passing through ovary.

Mount in (a) chloral hydrate and observe cluster crystals and

(b) phloroglucinol + HCl to observe xylem vessels, pericyclic fibres (lignified). (Ref. ACD)

3. Powder : Observe color, characteristic odor and taste. Mount in CH and train your eyes to recognize the minute pollen grains, the characteristic feature of clove powder. Observe pollen grains under HP also (PCD).

4. Extraction of volatile oil : 50 g of buds are taken and are subjected to steam distillation. The percentage of oil may vary from 14 to 21%. An interesting point to be noted here is while other essential oils remain at the top of the water distillate, clove oil being heavier than water goes to the bottom.

Chemical test: Few drops of essential oils are to be diluted in $CHCl_3$/toluene and on adding a few drop of $FeCl_3$ solution, a blue color is obtained due to the presence of eugenol, a phenol.

5. TLC of Clove oil : **Adsorbent:** Silica gel plate

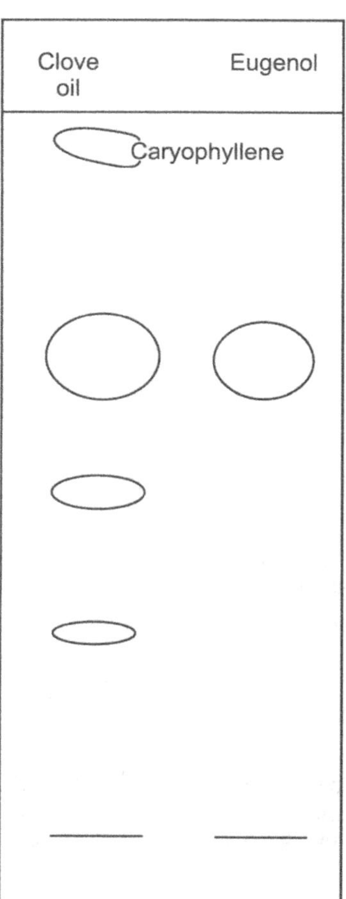

Solvent system:

Toluene: Ethyl acetate (93:7)

Application:

Clove oil (diluted in $CHCl_3$/ toluene 1:10) Eugenol to be applied as standard also diluted in 1: 30 ratio and 10 μl of each to be applied in band form.

Running distance: 10 cm

Drying:

Air drying for 15 min + in oven for 3-5 min.

Detection:

Cool, spray thoroughly with vanillin - H_2SO_4 reagent and heat the plate at 110°C for 5-10 min. under observation.

Record Rf values of eugenol and caryophyllene.

Eugenol (orange brown) approx. Rf value 0.7, Caryophyllene (reddish violet) runs to solvent front.

Record: Page I - 1; II - 2; III - 3; IV - 4,5

PYRETHRUM

Chrysanthemum cinerariiaefolium   Fam: **Compositae**

1. Morphology : Observe:
    (a) Entire flower head
    (b) LS of a flower head
    (c) Disc/tubular floret
    (d) Ray/ligulate floret

    Boil a few ray and disc florets in chloral hydrate solution, mount on a slide and observe under a dissection microscope. (Ref. SCD)

2. Powder : Note the color, odor and taste. Mount in CH and note the identifying characters as enlisted in PCD. Particularly observe the shape and nature of pollen grains and the T shaped trichomes.

    Record: Page I - 1 a, b, c, d; II – 2

SANTONICA/CINA

Artemisia cina   Fam: **Compositae**

1. Morphology : This is the smallest flower head known. Boil a few flower heads in CH solution, mount and observe the following:
    (a) Entire flower head
    (b) LS of a flower head (both under a dissection microscope)
    (c) Bract under a compound microscope (5x X LP) to observe bract cells, covering trichomes and glandular trichomes. (Ref. SCD)

2. Powder : Note the color, odor and taste. Mount in CH and note the identifying characters as enlisted in PCD. Particularly observe the shape and nature of pollen grains and the small worm shaped covering trichomes.

    (**Attention:** The fibres of blotting/filter paper which are likely to creep in, have similarity with COV. Tri. of cina but are more thicker and longer.)

    Record: Page I - 1 a, b, c; II - 2.

BARK DRUGS

General Instructions

1. Morphology : **Observe :**

      (a) Condition: fresh, dried etc.

      (b) Shape: flat, channelled, quill, double quill, compound quill, recurved etc.

      (c) Size: length, breadth, thickness.

      (d) Outer surface: color, striations, fissures, corrugations, lenticels, lichens, mosses etc.

      (e) Inner surface: color, characters like striations etc.

      (f) Fracture: short, fibrous etc.

      (g) Fractured surface: color; starchy, horny.

      (h) Odor and taste.

      Diagrams showing outer and inner surfaces

2. Microscopy : Dried samples are to be soaked atleast for 8-10 h. in water before taking sections/boiled in water for 30 min. While taking the TS of bark drugs, it is not the length of the bark piece that is important but it's thickness. All the tissues from the outer cork to the innermost secondary phloem tissues are to be seen in a proper section.

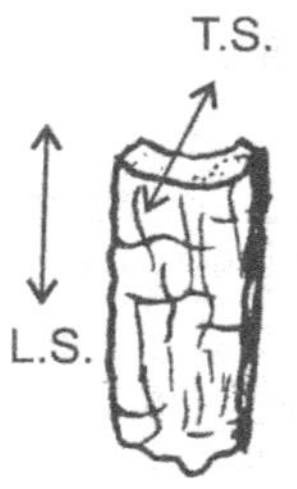

Unlike leaf sections, bark sections can be cut easily and can be boiled and cleared thoroughly in chloral hydrate solution. The lignified tissues like phloem fibres, pericyclic fibres, sclereids/stone cells are stained with phloroglucinol + Con. HCl mixture. Starch grains when present can be seen in a slide mounted in water and irrigated with dil. Iodine solution.

3. Powders : Note the color, odor and taste.

Mount in CH and observe the different types of crystals etc.

In a stained preparation observe lignified tissues, which form the basis for identifying and differentiating the various bark drugs. In a dil. Iodine stained preparation observe starch if and when present.

CASCARA

Rhamnus purshiana   Fam: **Rhamnaceae**

1. Morphology   :   Diagrams of outer surface and inner surface to be drawn. Refer SCD

2. Microscopy   :   In CH mount the phloem fibres and sclereids look yellowish.

Observe crystal sheath and cluster crystals.

In a stained slide observe the characteristic phloem fibres and sclereids. (ACD)

3. Powder   :   Note the color, odor and taste of the powder. In CH mount the powder takes yellow color throughout.

In a stained preparation observe the characteristic phloem fibres and sclereids. (PCD)

On addition of few drops of KOH solution to a powder sample on the slide, appearance of pink color confirms the presence of anthracene derivatives.

Chemical test: Borntrager's test (given under Senna) is to be performed.

4. TLC   :

Preparation of the extract:

1 g of powdered drug is heated with 10 ml of studies. methanol for 5 min, cooled and filtered. The filtrate is used for TLC studies.

Absorbent : Silica gel plate

Solvent system:

Ethyl acetate: MeOH: H_2O (100:13.5:10)

Application: In band form Cascara extract - 30 µl

Aloin (1% in MeOH) - 10 µl

Running distance: 10 to 12 cm.

Drying: Air drying for 15 min. and in oven for 10 min.

Detecton: Cool, spray with methanolic KOH solution and warm for 5 to 10 min. in oven.

Observe under UV and record the Rf value of aloin, chrysaloin, cascarosides CD and AB (if seen clearly)

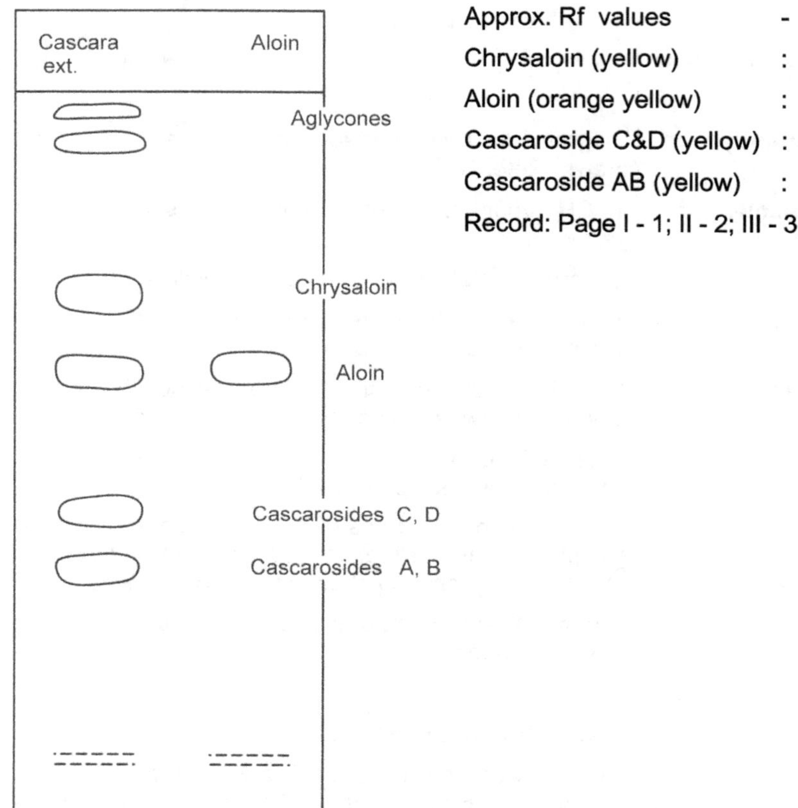

Approx. Rf values   -

Chrysaloin (yellow)   :   0.7

Aloin (orange yellow)   :   0.6

Cascaroside C&D (yellow) :   0.4

Cascaroside AB (yellow)   :   0.3

Record: Page I - 1; II - 2; III - 3; IV - 4.

CINCHONA

Cinchona species   Fam: **Rubiaceae**

1. Morphology   :   Observe the salient features of dried barks as indicated in SCD. Draw neat labelled diagrams in your record.

2. Microscopy   :   In chloralhydrate, mount and observe microsphenoidal cryst. In a stained preparation note the characteristic pink colored phloem fibres and absence of any type of stone cells. (ACD)

3. Powder   :   Note the color, odor and taste.

Observe the phloem fibres - their length and breadth and blunt ends. Compare these with those of Cassia. You should train your eyes to distinguish one from the other. (PCD)

4. Chemical tests: Thalleioquinn test - Refer SCD

For one another test, refer PCD and perform.

5. TLC   :   **Preparation of the extract:** Extract 1 g of bark powder with 5ml methanol containing a drop of ammonia on a water bath for 10min.at 60°C. Filter and take the filtrate for TLC studies.

Adsorbent: Silica gel plate

Solvent system:

Chloroform	:	Diethylamine (9:1)
Application	:	Apply in spot form
Cinchona extract	:	20 µl
Quinine Standard	:	10 µl
Quinidine Standard	:	10 µl
Cinchonine Standard	:	10 µl

(1% of test substances prepared in MeOH)

Running distance: 10 to 12 cm.

Drying: Plates are to be air dried for 15 min.

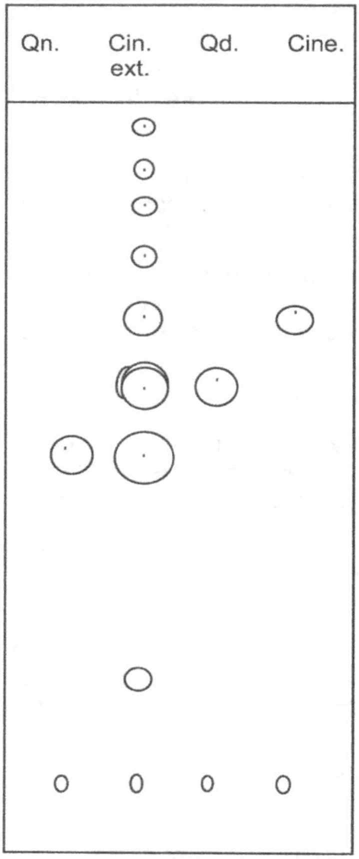

Qn.	Cin. ext.	Qd.	Cine.

Detection:

Spray thoroughly with 10% methanolic H_2SO_4. Heat the plate at 100 °C for 10 min. Observe under UV 365 nm (spots are not visible in the visual light).

Record the Rf values and appropriate colors in your journal.

Approx. Rf values of

Quinine (intense blue)	:	0.4-0.5
Quinidine (Blue)	:	0.5-0.6
Cinchonidine (violet)	:	0.5-0.6
Cinchonine (dark violet)	:	0.6-0.7

As quinidine overlaps cinchonidine, a violet tinge of cinchonidine is seen overlapping the bluish quinidine spot.

Record: Page I - 1; II - 2;

III - 3,4; IV - 5.

CINNAMON/CASSIA

Cinnamomum zeylanicum   Fam: **Lauraceae**
Cinnamomum cassia

These two species differ from one another in many aspects. However, the most important one C-zeylanicum is the inner bark whereas C.cassia is the entire bark. As a result, we do find significant microscopic differences. That apart, there are important chemical differences and these aspects will be touched at the appropriate places. What is available mostly in all the labs is the Cassia bark which is cheap hence Cassia will be taken up as the drug for practical.

1. Morphology : Observe the important features of both the species as given in SCD and draw neat diagrams in your record.

2. Mioroscopy : Dried bark pieces soaked for 24 h are given for taking sections. A CH mount will show minute acicular rephides either in the medullary ray cells or phloem parenchyma under HP. Water mount with a touch of iodine will show starch grains. A stained section will show sclereids, pericyclic fibres and the characteristic phloem fibres. The stone cells or the sclereids appear in band form and individually appear like U shaped. This again is very characteristic. (ACD)

3. Powder : Note the color, odor and taste. Observe the size and shape of the phloem fibres and try to differentiate from those of Cinchona powder. A stained preparation of the powder will show lignified fibres. Study the identifying characters as given in PCD.

4. Cassia oil : Note down the color, odor and taste of oil provided to you. Dilute 0.5 ml of Cassia oil in 5 ml alcohol, add 2 drops of ferric chloride solution and note the brown color due to the presence of cinnamaldehyde. Cinnamon oil however gives green color due to the combined presence of cinnamaldehyde and eugenol.

5. TLC of Cassia oil   :

Adsorbent; Silica gel plate.

Solvent system:

Toluene: ethyl acetate (93:7)

Application:

To be applied in band form.

Cassia oil diluted in toluene/chloroform in the proportion 1: 10 and cinnamaldehyde in the proportion 1:30; 10 µl of each is to be applied in the band form.

Running distance: 10 cm

Drying:

Air drying for 15 min. and in an oven for 3 to 5 min.

Detection:

Cool the plate, spray thoroughly with vanillin-H_2SO_4 reagent and heat at 110 °C for 5-10 min. under observation (till grey brown spots appear)

Caution: Avoid over heating.

Record Rf value of Cinnamaldehyde (Approx. 0.6-0.7) both standard and as well that from the Cassia oil. Reproduce the grey brown color in your record as seen in the visual light.

Record: Page I - 1; II - 2; III - 3,4; IV - 5.

KURCHI

Holarrhena antidysenterica   Fam: **Apocynaceae**

1. Morphology : Observe the diagnostic features of recurved bark pieces as given in SCD. Draw neat labelled sketches.

2. Microscopy : A thin CH mount will show rhomboidal Calcium oxalate crystals in parenchyma and also inside the sclereids.

A stained section shows bands of lignified sclereids. It is interesting to note the conspicuous absence of phloem fibres. A water mount with an iodine touch shows the presence of starch grains. (ACD)

3. Powder : Note the color, odor and taste. Observe the identifying characters as given in PCD. Observe both CH mounts and stained mounts.

4. TLC : **Preparation of the extract:**

Kurchi   Conessine
ext

Yellow background

1 g of the bark powder is taken in 10 ml methanol containing 1 or 2 drops of ammonia, heated on a water bath for 10 min., filtered and the filtrate used for TLC studies.

Adsorbent : Silica gel plate.

Solvent System:

Toluene/benzene): Ethyl acetate:

Diethylamine (7 : 2 :1)

Application: To be applied in band form

Kurchi extract: 20 µl

Conessine: 10 µl (0.5 mg in 5 ml methanol)

Running distance: 10 to 12 cm.

Drying:

Air drying for 15 min. and in oven for 3 to 5 min.

Detection:

Cool the plate and spray with Dragendorff's reagent. In the Kurchi extract 6 orange brown colored spots can be clearly seen. Note the Rf value of standard Conessine and that present in the extract (approx 0.8). The spots disappear after sometime. Therefore transfer the TLC results in your record directly. The spots do appear on spraying again.

Record: Page I - 1; II - 2; III - 3; IV - 4.

QUILLAIA

Quillaia saponaria   Fam: **Rosaceae**

1. Morphology : Observe the morphological characters of the inner bark as given in SCD, draw and describe the same in your journal.

2. Powder : Observe the color, odor and taste. Mount the powder in CH. Observe the groups of phloem fibres and try to differentiate these from those of Senna, Cascara and Licorice. Also observe the scattered calcium oxalate prisms. Note the absence of cork cells. Mount a stained section to observe the lignified phloem fibres.

3. Chemical Test : Shake a pinch of powder with 2 ml of water and see a copious persistent froth formed due to the presence of saponins.

Journal: Page I - 1; II – 2,3.

WOOD DRUG

QUASSIA

Picrasma excelsa   Fam: **Simarubaceae**

1. Morphology : The wood chips cut in various angles are available. Note and draw them as show in SCD.

2. Microscopy : Being a wood the histological aspects are studied by taking sections in three different perspectives i.e., TS, TLS & RLS (Refer ACD). Select a properly cut piece of the wood soaked in water for 24 h and note the different surfaces.

Wood being hard, it is possible to take thinnest possible sections. As usual in a CH mount, cal. oxalate prisms should be observed. In a stained mount, where all tissues take stain (being a wood), observe the vessels in different planes and so also the tracheids and wood fibres. Take care not to over stain the sections.

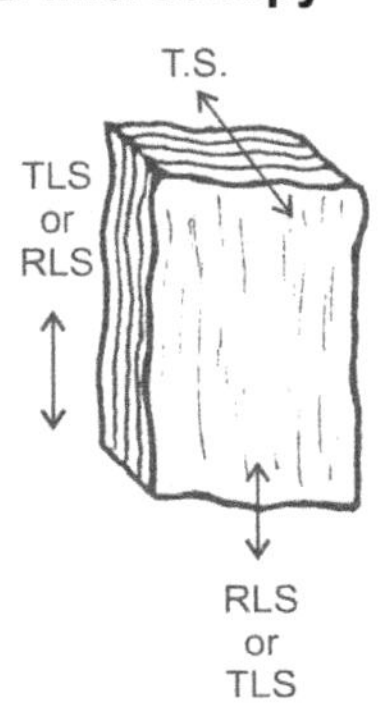

Try to differentiate the TLS from RLS. Note the nature of meduallary rays in different sections.

Display all the three stained sections under one and the same coverslip on a slide.

3. Powder : Observe color, odor and taste. Study the identifying characters as given in PCD.

Record: Page I - 1; II - 2; III - 3.

ROOTS & RHIZOME DRUGS

The dried roots and rhizomes are to be soaked overnight in water to make them soft, so that sections can be taken easily. Hard and thick roots like those of Rauwolfia are to be soaked for 24 h. In case of thick samples, a portion of the section will suffice. Roots generally contain starch grains, therefore sections and powders are to be mounted in water and irrigated with Iodine solution to study the nature of the grains.

ACONITE

Aconitum species   Fam: **Ranunculaceae**

1. Morphology : Morphology of the various market samples (SCD).

2. TS : It is advisable to take a complete section at the lower tapering end in order to study the nature of the cambium ring. Study the various tissues as given in ACD and record them.

3. Powder : Note down the color, odor and taste of the powder. Prepare three slides (CH, stained, I_2) and note down the diagnostic characters, especially the characteristic stone cells.

4. TLC : **Preparation of the Extract:** Take 1 g of the powder in 10 ml methanol, add 2-3 drops of ammonia soln. and heat on a water bath for 5 min. Cool, filter and use the filtrate for TLC studies.

Adsorbent: Silica gel plate.

Solvent System:

Toluene/Benzene: Ethyl acetate:

Diethylamine (7:2:1). To be more precise take only 21 + 6 + 3 = 30 ml of solvent mixture and saturate the chamber for atleast 1 h.

Application: To be applied in band form. Aconite extract: 30 μl

Running distance: 1·0 or 12 cm.

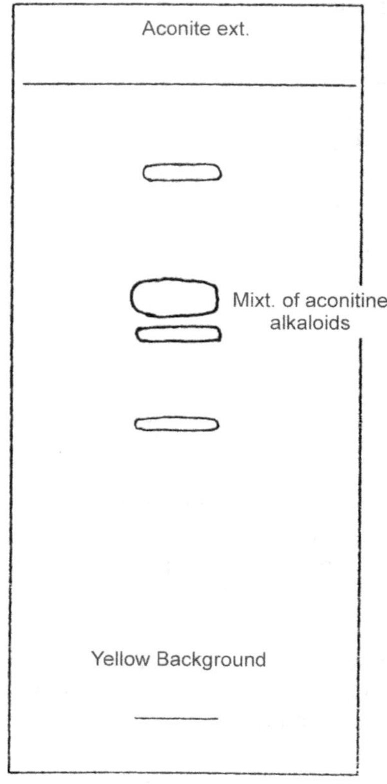

Drying: After removing plates from jar they are to be air dried for 15 min. and then in an oven for 5 min. (to ensure complete drying).

Detection: Cool the plate and spray with Dragendorff 's reagent.

Observe two prominent orange colored spots in the Rf range of 0.6 and 0.7 which represent the mixture of aconitine alkaloids. Record the TLC plate with proper color immediately.

Record: Page I - 1; II - 2; III - 3; IV - 4.

GENTIAN

Gentiana lutea   Fam: **Gentianaceae**

Source, morphological descriptions, active constituents and uses (ruled page).

1. Morphology : On the unruled page: Salient external features of dried roots to be drawn. (Ref. SCD)

2. Powder : Observe the color, odor and taste. Mount the powder in CH, and also stain a preparation of the powder. Note the nature of xylem vessels and try to differentiate these from those of Podophyllum (Ref.PCD)

Record: Page I - 1, 2.

IPECAC

Cephaelis ipecacuanha/C. acuminata   Fam: **Rubiaceae**

1. Morphology : Note the important features as given in SCD and draw suitable diagrams in the journal.

2. TS : Take entire sections of the roots (soaked over night) and mount in CH, Phloroglucinol + HCl and also in Iodine soln. and observe the tissues as in ACD. In CH mount, observe bundles of acicular raphides. In the stained section observe lignified wood elements and starch in the Iodine preparation. Draw a neat diagram in your record.

3. Powder : Observe the color, odor and taste of the powder. Here again make three different mounts as mentioned above and study all the identifying characters (PCD) and draw the same in the journal.

4. TLC : **Preparationof extract:** 1 g of the powdered Ipecac is warmed with 5 ml of MeOH containing few drops of ammonia soln., on water bath at 60 °C for 5 min. Cool the mixture, filter and use the filtrate for TLC studies.

Adsorbent: Silica gel plates

Solvent System:

Toluene/Benzene: Ethyl acetate: Diethylamine (7: 2: 1). Take 30 ml of this mixture in the proportion of (21 +6+3). Saturate the jar for 3-4 h.

Compounds	In visual light	Under UV	Rf value (approx)
Emetine	Yellow	Yellow	0.7
Cephaeline	Brownish	Light bluish	0.5
Psychotrine	Light brown	Light blue	0.06
O'methyl psychotrine	Light yellow	Light yellow	0.6

5. TLC :

Application:

All in band form. Ipecac extract: 30 µl

Emetine: 10 µl (1% in MeOH soln.)

Cephaeline: 10 µl.

(1% in MeOH soln.)

Running distance: 10-12 cm.

Drying: After the run, the plates are to be air dried completely in an oven for 3-5 min.

Detection:

1. Spray the plate with I_2-CHCl$_3$ reagent (0.5% I_2 in CHCl$_3$) and heat again for 10 min at 60 °C.

2. Observe under UV 365 nm as well as in visual light and note down the colors of Emetine, Cephaeline, Psychotrine and O' methyl psychotrine.

3. Record the Rf values and draw in your journal with the help of proper colors.

(**Note:** With well saturated chambers Rf of Emetine is above 0.5 and without proper saturation less than 0.5).

Journal: Page I - 1; II - 2; III - 3; IV - 4.

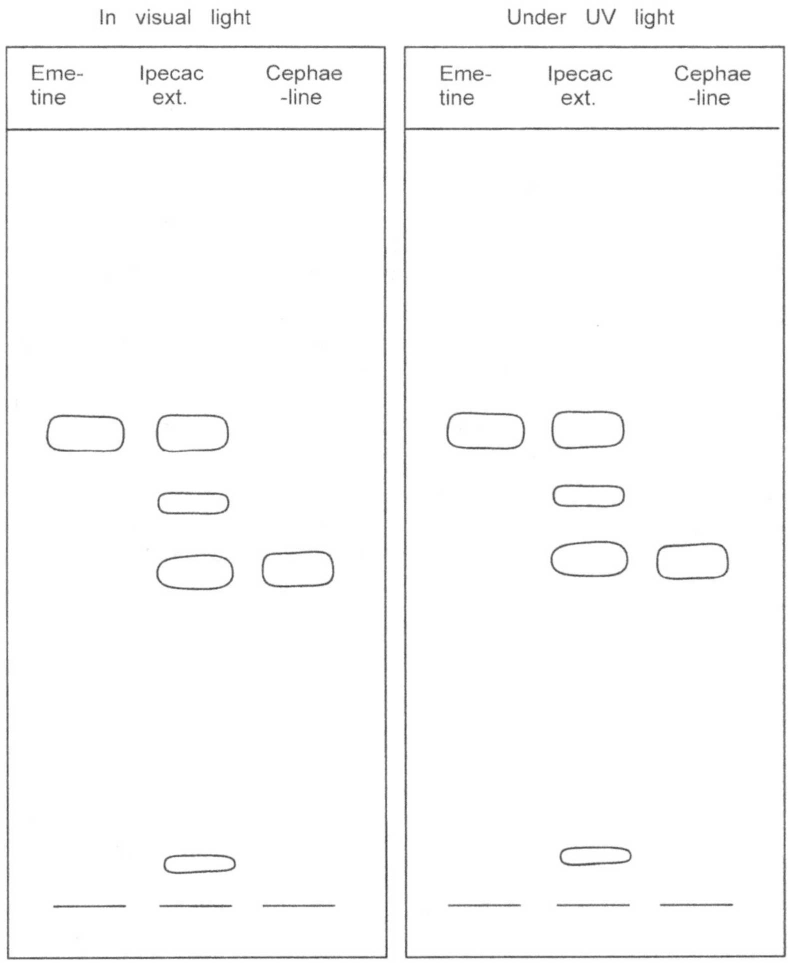

In   visual   light
Under   UV   light
Eme-
tine
Ipecac
ext.
Cephae
-line
Eme-
tine
Ipecac
ext.
Cephae
-line

LICORICE

Glycyrrhiza glabra   Fam: **Leguminosae**

1. Morhology : Observe the different samples namely thin roots, thick roots, stolons and study the external character as given in SCD. Sweet taste and the yellowish colored transverse surface help to identify the drug easily.

2. Microscopy : Take TS of either a root or stolon which is already soaked. With thick samples, a portion will suffice. Mount the sections as usual in CH, Phloroglucinol + HCl, dil. Iodine soln. (water mount and then with I_2 to be irrigated). Study the tissues as given in ACD. The difference between stolon and root is to be noted.

3. Powder : Prepare 3 slides as usual and observe the diagnostic characters as given in PCD. CH will turn yellow when licorice powder is mounted. Observe carefully the yellowish colored crystal sheath/fibres.

4. TLC : **Preparation of drug extract:**

1. Shake 1 g of licorice powder with 20 ml $CHCl_3$ for 20 to 30 min. and filter. Evaporate the filtrate completely and dissolve the residue in 2 ml of $CHCl_3$ + MeOH (1:1) mixture.

2. Heat the chloroform extracted powder under reflux for 1 h with 30 ml of 0.5 N H_2SO_4. Cool the mixture and shake with 20 ml of chloroform twice. Combime chloroform extracts, dry over Na_2SO_4 (anhydrous), filter and evaporate completely. Dissolve the residue in 2 ml $CHCl_3$ + MeOH (1:1) mixture. Again we have here now a chloroform extract but after hydrolysis.

4. TLC : **Adsorbent:** Silica gel plate

Solvent System:

Chloroform: Methanol (95:5)

Application:

To be applied in band form.

Chloroform extract : 20 μl

Chloroform extract after hydrolysis: 20 μl

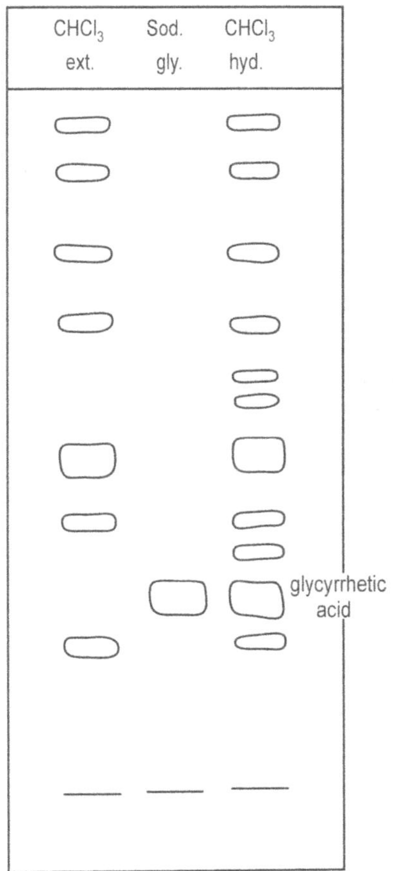

Glycyrrhetic acid/Sodium glycyr-rhizinate (0.1% in MeOH):

10 µl (if the test sample is available).

Running distance: 10-12 cm.

Drying:

Plates are air dried for 15 min.

Detection:

1. Spray thoroughly with anisaldehyde - H_2SO_4 reagent.

2. Heat at 100 °C for 10-15 min. under observation.

3. Observe the glycyrrhetic acid (red - violet) spot in the hydrolyzed extract.

Record Rf of glycyrrhetic acid (approx. 0.25) and display the chart with proper colors in your record.

Record: Page I – 1; II - 2; III - 3; IV - 4.

RAUWOLFIA

Rauwolfia serpentina   Fam: **Apocynaceae**

1. Morphology   :   Observe the thick as well as thin roots of Rauwolfia and note the salient features as given in SCD. Draw neat labelled diagrams.

2. Microscopy   :   As the central wood portion is very hard, the thin roots are preferred for taking TS. The roots are to be soaked in water for 24 h. Take sections carefully (good many chances of your fingers getting cut!!) with the bark intact, mount and observe the important characters as given in SCD.

In CH mount: see twin prisms. In the stained section: see lignified cork/stratified cork, lignified wood and medullary rays.

In Iodine mount: starch grains with a characteristic hilum.

Draw a neat labelled diagrams in the record as given in ACD.

3. Powder   :   Observe the color, odor and taste of the powder. As usual make three slides using the three different mounts and study all the identifying characters (PCD).

4. TLC   :   **Preparation of the extract:**

Add few drops of ammonia to 5 ml MeOH and to this now add 1 g of Rauwolfia powder and heat on a water bath for 10 min. at 60 $^{\circ}$C. Filter and use the filtrate for TLC studies.

Adsorbent: Silica gel plates

Solvent System: Toluene/Benzene:

Ethyl acetate: Diethylamine (7:2:1). Take 30 ml

(21+6+3) mixture in the jar and saturate atleast for 1 h.

Application: Applied in band form

Rauwolfia extract: 20 μl.

Reserpine: 10 μl.

(0.5% methanolic solution)

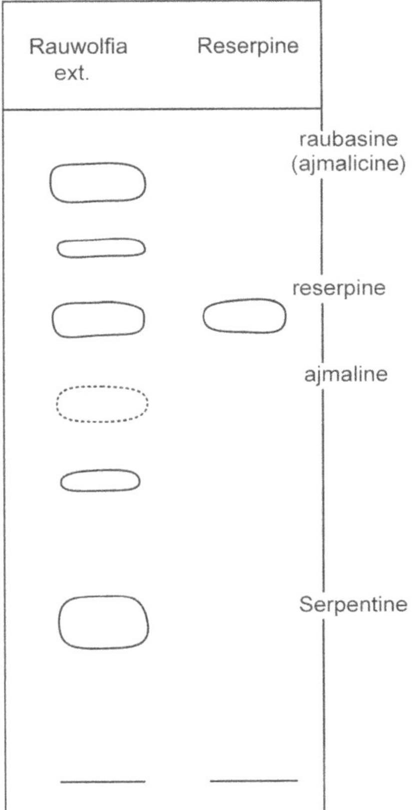

Running distance: 12 Cm.

Drying: The plates are to be air dried for 15-20 min. and in oven at 100 °C for 5-10 min.

Detection:

1. No spots are visible in the visual light.

2. Cool the plate and observe under UV 365 nm.

3. Mark the entire spots with the help of the needle or a pointer under UV.

4. Note down the colors of Reserpine (fluoresces light greenish yellow) and Serpentine (fluoresces dark blue).

5. To detect Ajmaline, spray carefully the lower 2/3rd portion of the plate with conc. HNO_3. Ajmaline is seen as a red spot in visual light.

6. Calculate the Rf values of Reserpine (0.65-0.75), Ajmaline (0.5-0.6) and Serpentine (0.3-0.35)

Reproduce the plate in your record with properly colored spots.

Note:

1. Handle HNO_3 carefully while spraying.

2. Unless the plates are properly dried in oven, the spots will not fluoresce.

Journal: Page I - 1; II - 2: III - 3, IV - 4.

GINGER

Zingiber officinale   Fam: **Zingiberaceae**

1. Morphology : Observe both fresh as well as dried samples of rhizomes. Draw neat labelled sketches in the record and refer SCD.

2. Microscopy : Take TS of fresh rhizomes and mount in CH. Observe yellowish oleoresin cells.

Phloroglucinol + HCl - lignified tissues (???)

Iodine water mount - starch grains. Draw and describe the TS in the record (Ref. ACD).

3. Powder : Observe as usual color, odor and taste. Make three slides, one in CH, the other in Phloroglucinol + HCl and the third in Iodine-water. Study all the characters by referring to PCD. Measurement of starch grains may will be attempted here as these resemble somewhat those of potato. Note the differences.

Essential oil of Ginger : **Extraction:** Take about 100 g of fresh Ginger rhizomes and cut them into small pieces. Distil the oil and find out the yield (... %).

4. TLC : **Adsorbent:** Silica gel plate.

Solvent System: 93:7 ratio of Toluene/Benzene: Ethyl acetate. Chamber to be saturated atleast for 1 h.

Application: Ginger oil to be diluted in chloroform or toluene in 1:10 proportion. 10 μl is to be applied in band form.

Reference standards, if available like - Zingiberene, Zingiberol etc. and these also to be diluted like the oil.

Running distance: 10 to 12 cm.

Drying: After the run, plates are to be air dried for 15-20 min. and in oven for 5 min.

Detection: Cool the plate, spray thoroughly with vanillin-H_2SO_4 reagent, heat at 110 $^{\circ}$C for 5-10 min. under observation. Record Rf values of known

compounds in visual light. Reproduce the TLC plate in your record book with proper colors.

Journal: Page I- 1; II 2; III - 3; IV - 4.

RHUBARB

Rheum emodi   Fam: **Polygonaceae**

1. Morphology : The market samples vary in size and shape. Observe the morphological characters of different samples carefully. Draw neat labelled diagrams (Ref.SCD).

2. Powder : Mount the powder in CH - large cluster crystals are characteristic identifying characters. Also chloral hydrate turns yellow. In a stained preparation, note the unlignified vessels. Thus, vessels of Gentian and Podophyllum can be distinguished. In an Iodine - water mount observe, starch grains.

Chemical test: Powder + KOH soln. = Red color (Presence of anthracene derivatives).

3. TLC : Preparation of the drug extract (hydrolyzed extract): Take 50 mg of powdered drug and heat it on a water bath for 15 min. in a mixture of 3 ml of water and 1 ml of con. HCl. Cool the mixture and extract with 25 ml ether. Separate ethereal layer, dry over anhyd.Na_2SO_4 and filter. Reduce the soln. almost to dryness under vacuum. Dissolve this in 0.5 ml ether and use for TLC studies.

Adsorbent: Silica gel plate

Solvent System: Petroleum ether (40°- 60°):

Ethyl acetate: HCOOH free of water (75:25:1).

Saturate the chamber properly.

Application: Rhubarb extract 30 µl.

Running distance: 12cm

Reference compounds like Rheum - emodin (1% soln. in ether): 10 µl

Drying:

Air dry for 15 min. and in an oven for 5-10 min. at 100 °C.

Detection:

1. Observe under UV (365 nm).

2. Expose the plate to ammonia vapour and observe in visual light.

Journal: Page I - 1; II - 2; III – 3

Compound	Color Under UV	Color after exposure to NH_3 in VL	Approx. Rf value
Chrysophenol	Yellow	Yellowish red	0. 9
Physcion	Yellow	Yellowish red	0.85
Rheum emodin	Yellow	orange red	0.5
Rhein	Yellow	Yellowish red	0.4
Aloe-emodin	Yellow	orange red	0.35

Under UV 365 nm

After exposure to ammonia

PODOPHYLLUM

Podophyllum hexandrum/P. emodi   Fam: **Berberidaceae**

1. Morphology : Observe and record the diagnostic morphological characters of dried rhizomes and roots (Ref. SCD). Draw neat labelled diagrams in the journal.

2. Microscopy : Take thin TS of both rhizomes and roots which are soaked overnight. The rhizome being tortuous, it is difficult to get all the vascular bundles cut transversely in a section. Present only a portion of the rhizome section wherein vascular bundles are cut transversely. It is very easy to take a thin and complete section of the roots. Mount both sections separately in a) CH mount, b) Iodine mount and c) a stained section. Study the tissues as given in ACD and draw neat labelled diagrams of both in your journal.

3. Powder : Study the powder carefully and observe the important identifying characters from PCD. Illustrate these in your record.

Adulterant: Observe the rhizomes of **Ainsliaea latifolia**, Fam: Asteraceae which is also sold as Podophyllum in the Indian Market. Note the wooly fibres at the base of the stem by which it differs from **P. hexandrum** morphologically.

4. TLC : **Preparation of the extract:** 1 g of powdered drug is taken in 10 ml of ethanol, extracted for 15 min, filtered and the filtrate used for TLC studies.

Adsorbent: Silica gel plates.

Solvent System: Two systems are to be used one after the other.

$CHCl_3$: MeOH (9:1)

$CHCl_3$: Acetone (65:35)

Application: Applied in band form

Phodophyllum extract: 30 μl.

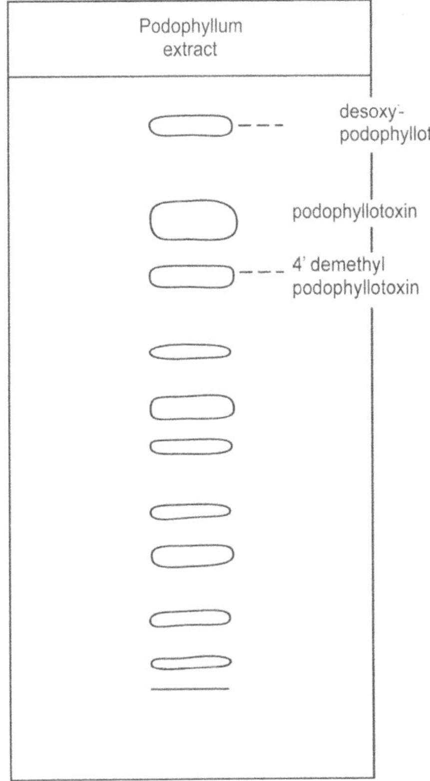

Running distance: Two steps are involved. Run up to 5 cm in $CHCl_3$: MeOH (9:1). Air dry for 15 min. and then again run upto a distance of 15 cm, in $CHCl_3$: Acetone (65:35).

Drying: Plates are air dried for 15- 20 min (in the oven for 5 min. if necessary).

Detection: Spray carefully with Con. H_2SO_4 and heat for 5 to 10 min. at 100 °C.

Observation: Observe the greyish brown spots in visual light and record Rf values (0.8) of Podophyllotoxin. Illustrate the TLC chart in your record.

Journal: Page I - 1; II - 2; III - 2; IV - 3; V - 4.

VALERIAN

Valeriana wallichii   Fam: **Valerianaceae**

1. Morphology : Observe the salient features of both root and rhizome available in dried condition. The drug can easily be identified due to its characteristic stinking odor. Draw neat labelled diagrams in the journal (Refer: SCD)

2. TS : As both rhizomes and roots are important, the microscopic studies of both parts must be studied. The rhizomes are to be soaked overnight, but roots being thin and delicate soaking for one hour will suffice. The roots being thin, it may be difficult to hold and take sections. Hence potato pieces may be used as pith to support so that sections can be taken easily. Here again mount the sections in the usual three different mounts and study the tissues by following ACD. Make a special note of the tissues containing the active principles in both.

3. Powder : Note the color, odor and taste.

Mount the powder as well in the three different mounts and study the identifying characters as per PCD.

Journal: Page I - 1; II - 2 (rhizome); III - 2(root); IV - 3.

SEED DRUGS

For seed drugs, you have to observe their shape, size, external surface, any outgrowths, the presence and position of hilum, micropyle, raphe etc. Similarly in TS one has to concentrate broadly on three tissues only- testa, endosperm and cotyledons of the embryo. While the reserve food content in the earlier drugs has been starch grains in general, here we have instead aleurone grains (proteinaceous in nature) and fixed oils in the form of globules in endosperm and cotyledons. However in some cases we have one more nutritive tissue derived from nucellus namely perisperm which surrounds endosperm and is starchy in nature. Details of these tissues will be dealt under the concerned drugs.

ISAPGOL

Plantago ovata   Fam: **Plantaginaceae**

1. Morphology : The seeds being very small, a hand lens may be used to observe the macroscopic characters. Draw magnified diagrams of both surfaces and write the magnification with the sub titles (Ref.SCD).

2. TS : Seeds are not to be soaked in water. Due to the presence of mucilage when in contact with water, the seeds swell up and become slippery. Keep the dry seeds on the glass slide and cut thin sections on the slide only. Mount the sections as mentioned below:

In CH: Just warm the sections enough to remove the air bubbles. Over boiling will displace the cotyledons from their place. (Your section is complete only when there is an epidermal layer) **In Phloroglucinol + HCl:** Only the minute xylem vessels of the vascular bundles take up the stain. **In Ruthenium Red:** Add few drops of freshly prepared ruthenium red soln. to the dry section on the glass slide, put the coverslip and observe under the microscope. The epidermal layer swells up and takes red color due to mucilage. Observe the tissues and draw labelled sketches in the record (Ref. ACD).

3. Powder   :

Mount the powder in

(a)   CH mount

(b)   In Ruthenium red soln. Epidermal fragments take up pink color.

(c)   In water mount – epidermis swells up and is seen clearly.

Draw and label the characters as given in PCD.

Isapghul husk: This is the commercial Isapghul. Observe its nature and take note of the market preparations containing Isapghul husk (Nature care, Softovac etc.)

4. Swelling factor   :

This is a parameter to judge the quality of the drug. The principle behind this experiment is the presence of mucilage which absorbs water and swells. The swelling of the seed can be determined quantitatively by what is called as swelling factor. Take 1 g of Isapgol seeds in a 25 ml stoppered measuring cylinder. Add 20 ml water, shake occasionally during the first 23 h and leave it undisturbed for one more hour. The increase in volume is the swelling factor. For quality seeds it is between 10 to 14 and for the husk it is around 20.

Journal: Page I – 1; II – 2; III - 3, 4.

LINSEED

Linum usitatissimum   Fam: **Linaceae**

1. Morphology : Observe the seeds using a hand lens and draw magnified diagrams in your record (Ref. SCD).

2. TS : Do not soak the seeds in water for a long time. Just before taking the sections dip the seeds in water and then take sections. Otherwise, here again like Isaphgol the seeds swell up due to mucilage. Take entire sections and mount the sections in:

(a) CH: Do not boil too much in CH. Otherwise, testa and endosperm get separated.Take care while putting the coverslip also.

(b) Phloroglucinol + HCl: the sclerenchyma layer takes up the stain.

(c) Ruthenium red: Pick up a fresh section and mount in Ruthenium red soln. Put the coverslip and observe under a microscope. The epidermal layer takes up the red stain due to the presence of mucilage. (Ref. ACD for diagrams and reproduce the same in your record).

3. Powder : Observe the color, odor and taste.

Mount the powder in CH and also in Phloroglucinol + HCl (sclerenchyma fibres take up the stain). In Ruthenium Red soln. only the epidermal fragments take the pink color (Ref. PCD for diagrams).

When linseed powder is wrapped in a piece of paper, the paper shows oily marks due to the presence of fixed oils in the seed. This also gives some clue for the presence of linseed powder in a mixture.

Journal: Page I - 1; II - 2; III - 3.

STROPHANTHUS

Strophanthus gratus /S. kombe   Fam: **Apocynaceae**

1. Morphology : Study carefully the morphological features of both **S. Kombe** and **S. gratus** seeds (if both are available). Note that most of the seeds sold under the name of Strophanthus in Indian Market are the seeds of Kurchi (They can easily be identified by color and by studying the microscopy. The TS of Kurchi seeds show convoluted cotyledons). Draw labelled diagrams in the record Ref. SCD).

2. Powder : Mount the powder in CH as well as in Phloroglucinol + HCl. Note the differences in the seeds of the two species by observing the presence or absence of lignified trichomes. Also try to differentiate these trichomes (when present) from those of Nux vomica (Ref: PCD)

Journal: Page I - 1, 2.

COFFEE

Coffea arabica   Fam: **Rubiaceae**

In this drug for obvious reasons we study only the powder and TLC.

1. Powder : Observe color, odor and taste. Mount the powder in CH. Remember that you gave to boil the powder preparation repeatedly till it gets cleared. In the Phloroglucinol + HCl mount, the lignified sclereids appear pink.

2. TLC : Refer Tea. (page no.23)

Journal: Page I - 1; II - 2.

NUX VOMICA

Strychnos nuxvomica   Fam: **Loganiaceae**

1. Morphology	:	Study the external features of the seeds. Take a longitudinal section (LS) of the seed and observe specially the cotyledons. Refer SCD and draw neat labelled diagrams.
2. TS	:	Take TS of a portion of the seed and observe the tissues as follows:

   (a) **In CH mount:** Handle sections carefully while transferring from watch glass to the slide. The tips of the trichomes get separated. Present a slide with entire trichomes intact.

   (b) **In Phloroglucinol + HCl mount:** The lignified trichomes take red color.

   (c) **In Iodine soln.:** When fresh and thin sections are observed under a microscope (first under LP objective and later HP objective), fine proto-plasmic strands between the endosperm cells are seen. These are called as 'Plasmodesmata'. Refer ACD and draw a neat labelled TS.

3. Powder : Observe color, odor and taste (take care, a deadly poisonous drug).

Mount the powder both in CH and also in Phloroglucinol + HCl. Try to differentiate the lignified trichomes of this from those of **Strophanthus kombe.**

4. TLC Studies : **Preparation of the extract:**

Powdered drugs containing fixed oils are to be first defatted with petroleum ether. Take 1 g of the defatted powder in 9.5 ml MeOH and 0.5 ml ammonia mixture. Extract for 10 min. on a steam bath. Cool, filter and use the filtrate for TLC studies.

Adsorbent: Silica gel plate.

Solvent System: Toluene/Benzene:

Ethyl acetate: Diethylamine (7: 2;1). For practical purposes take only 30 ml (21+6+3) in a jar. Chamber needs saturation for 1 h.

Application: To be applied in band form.

Nux vomica extract: 20 μl

Strychnine (1% MeOH soln.): 10 μl

Brucine (1% MeOH soln.): 10 μl

Running distance: 10 cm.

Drying: Air drying for 15-20 min. and in an oven for 3 to 5 min.

Detection: Cool the plate, spray with Dragendorff's reagent. Orange brown colored spots appear and fade away gradually. The plate may therefore be sprayed again, if necessary. Reproduce the TLC chart in your record with proper colors. Approx. range of Rf value of strychnine and brucine are 0.55 to 0.6 and 0.4 to 0.45 respectively.

Caution: Wash your hands thoroughly after the practical work.

Journal: Page I - 1; II - 2; III - 3; IV - 4.

FRUIT DRUGS

To observe the morphological peculiarities of some small fruits, one may here again use a hand lens. The stalk of the fruit or its point of attachment or its scar, the remains of calyx or stigma at the apex and the number of seeds in a fruit are all significant points worth noting. Unlike other fruits Umbelliferous fruits display certain characteristic features. Magnified sketches are to be drawn in the record to show all these characters.

The microscopy of the fruits reveals not only all the earlier studied characters of the seeds like testa, endosperm and sometimes cotyledons or embryo region but also in addition a new tissue collectively called as pericarp surrounding the testa, based on which tissue one can differentiate a fruit and a seed. Pericarp again is divided into three layers, namely the outer epicarp, the middle mesocarp and the inner endocarp. Some of these layers in some of the fruit drugs are very characteristic. In case of Umbelliferous fruits, isolation of the tissue containing the essential oil - the vittae- is also an important exercise to be carried out in the lab.

Powders of Umbelliferous drugs show certain common characters like fragments of vittae, parquetry layer of endocarp etc.

CAPSICUM

Capsicum annuum   Fam: **Solanaceae**

1. Morphology   :   Observe the dried fruits. Take a longitudinal section of the fruit. Observe, draw and label (Ref: SCD).

2. Powder   :   Color, odor and taste to be noted. Mount the powder in CH and observe and then make a preparation in Phloroglucinol + HCl. Note and illustrate in your record all the diagnostic characters given in PCD.

Journal: Page I - 1,2.

CARAWAY

Carum carvi   Fam: **Umbelliferae**

1. Morphology   :   Observe carefully the morphological characters of entire cremocarp and mericarp. Study the characters so as to differentiate from those of Fennel. Draw neat labelled diagrams as given in SCD.

2. Powder   :   Observe color, odor and taste. Mount the powder both in CH and as well in Phloroglucinol + HCl. Carefully observe the sclereids and fragments of vittae as given in PCD.

Caraway oil: Find out the percentage of oil in 50 g of Caraway fruits by steam distillation method.

3. TLC of Caraway oil:

Adsorbent: Silica gel plate.

Solvent System:

Toluene/Benzene: Ethyl acetate (93: 7) but then take 30 ml (27.9 + 2.1) mixture in a jar and saturate atleast for one hour.

Application: Applied as spots Caraway oil (distilled): 10 μl (1:10 dilution in Toluene/ $CHCl_3$) Caraway oil (market sample if available): 10 μl (dilution same as above) Carvone: 10 μl (1:30 dilution in Toluene/ $CHCl_3$)

Running distance: 10 cm.

Drying: The plate is to be air dried for 15 to 20 min. and in an oven for 3 to 5 min.

Detection: Cool and spray with Vanillin - H_2SO_4 reagent thoroughly and heat at 110 °C for 5-10 min. under observation. When raspberry (red violet) spots appear, take out the plate from the oven. Do not over heat the plate.

Illustrate the TLC chart in the journal and use proper colors. Carvone - approx. Rf value is 0.6 to 0.7.

Journal: Page I - 1 & 2; II - 3.

CORIANDER

Coriandrum sativum   Fam: **Umbelliferae**

1. Morphology : With the help of a magnifying glass or a hand lens, carefully observe the entire cremocarp. Split the fruit into 2 halves and observe the 2 surfaces of a mericarp, especially the nature of primary and secondary ridges on the dorsal surface. Draw magnified diagrams in the journal and label the parts as shown in SCD.

2. TS : Use fruits soaked overnight for taking section. Take TS of the entire cremocarps with carpophore intact. Very often the mericarps get separated while mounting on the slide or while staining. In such cases present complete section of a mericarp with carpophore intact and so also 2 vittae on the commisural surface. If the sections are taken at the upper one third portion, TS of embryo will also be seen in the central portion of the endosperm.

Mount and observe the sections in CH mount: Stain thereafter as usual with phloroglucinol + HCl. Note the lignified tissues like sclerenchymatous fibres of the mesocarp, vascular elements, carpophore etc. For more than one reason (small fruit, difficult to hold, sclerenchymatous mesocarp etc.) it is difficult to take a TS of Coriander. As a result you are likely to end up with thick or oblique sections. An oblique section can easily be identified by looking at the obliquely cut vittae on the commisural surface and the uneven lining of testa on the dorsal surface. Observe the various tissues as given in ACD and draw the diagram in the record.

3. Powder : Observe color, odor and taste. Mount in CH and also in Phloroglucinol + HCl and observe the important identifying characters as indicated in PCD. Draw neat labelled diagrams.

4. Distillation of
   Coriander oil :

Take 100 g of Coriander fruits and distil the volatile oil by steam distillation. Find out the percentage yield and use the same oil for TLC studies.

5. TLC of Coriander oil:

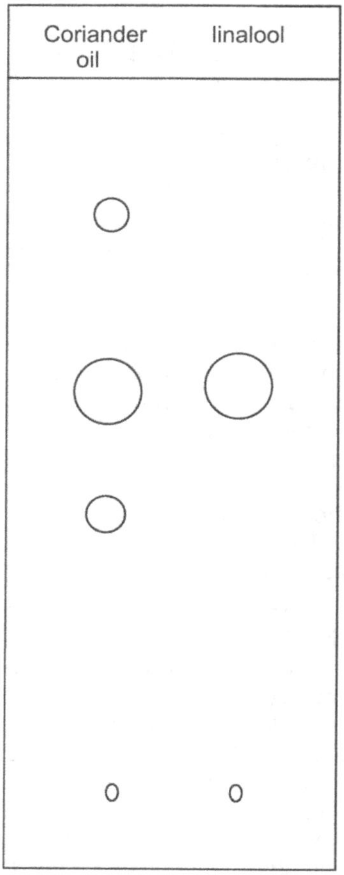

<table>
<tr><td>

Coriander oil   linalool

(TLC plate diagram with spots)

</td><td>

Adsorbent: Silica gel plate.

Solvent System:

Toluene/Benzene: Ethyl acetate (93:7). Take 30 ml (27.9 + 2.1) of the mixture in a jar, saturate for one hour.

Application: Spots or band form. Coriander oil: 10 μl (1:10 dilution in Toluene or Chloroform)

Linalool: 10 μl (1:30 dilution in Toluene or Chloroform).

Running distance: 10 cm

Drying:

Plates are to be air dried for 15-20 min. and in an oven for 3 to 5 min.

Detection:

Spray the plate thoroughly with Vanillin - H_2SO_4 reagent, heat at 110 $^{\circ}$C for 5 to 10 min. under observation till grey blue spots appear.

Record Rf values of Linalool (approx. 0.5-0.6) in visual light and reproduce a TLC chart with proper colors in your record.

Caution: Do not overheat the plate.

Journal: Page I - 1; II - 2; III - 3; IV - 4 & 5.

</td></tr>
</table>

FENNEL

Foeniculum vulgare   Fam: **Umbelliferae**

1. Morphology : Study the macroscopic features of an entire cremocarp and mericarp with the help of a magnifying glass. Note the differences between Fennel and Caraway. Draw and label (Ref.SCD).

2. TS : Overnight soaked fruits are used for taking sections. Take thin and complete sections of entire cremocarps. Mount the sections:

(a) In CH and observe under microscope

(b) In Phloroglucinol + HCl. Observe the lignified tissues taking up the stain (vascular bundles with reticulate parenchyma, raphe, carpophore etc.). Here again you are likely to take oblique sections. Check your sections whether oblique or not by observing all the 6 vittae of a mericarp.

Study the various tissues as given in ACD and draw a neat labelled diagram in the record.

3. Powder : Color, odor and taste are to be noted. Mount the powder in CH and study the characters. Also in a stained section observe the lignified reticulate parenchyma fragments scattered and also in association with the vascular strands. Study the powder characters as in PCD and illustrate the same in your record.

4. Isolation of vittae : Vitta is the most important character of Umbelliferous fruits as this tissue contains the active constituent namely the essential oil. To isolate these, boil few fennel fruits in 5% soln. of KOH or NaOH till they become soft. Take one fruit on a glass slide and tease it longitudinally with a pair of needles to separate brownish colored vittae from the adhering tissue. Remove the unwanted tissues and retain an entire vitta on the slide. Add CH, put coverslip and observe under LP objective. Sketch the same in the practical journal.

5. Fennel Oil : Take 50 g of fennel fruits and distil the oil in a steam distillation apparatus. Find out the percentage yield. The oil can be used for TLC purposes.

6. TLC of Fennel oil:

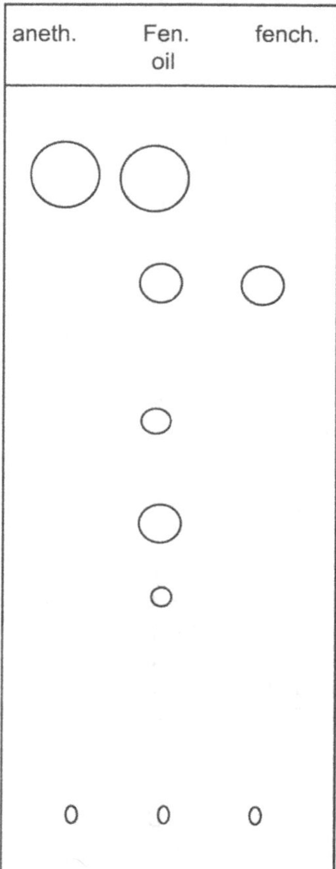

Adsorbent: Silica gel plate.

Solvent System:

Toluene/ Benzene: Ethyl acetate (93:7). Take 30 ml (27.9 + 2.1) mixture in a jar. Saturate the chamber for one hour.

Application: All in spot form. Fennel oil (distilled): 10 µl (1:10 dilution in Toluene/ $CHCl_3$)

Fennel oil (market sample if available) 10 µl (same dilution as above)

Anethole: 10 µl

(1:30 dilution in $CHCl_3$ / Toluene)

Fenchone: 10 µl

(dilution same as above)

Running distance: 10 to 12 cm

Drying: Air drying for 15-20 min. and in an oven for 5 min.

Detection:

1. Spray the plates first with 20% ethanolic soln. of Phosphomolybdic acid and heat at 110 °C for 5 to 10 min. under observation. Anethole spots appear bluish.

2. To locate Fenchone, cool the plate and spray again with $KMnO_4$ - H_2SO_4 reagent (spray carefully) and heat at 110 °C for 5-10 min. under observation. Fenchone spots appear bluish (do not overheat).

Observation: All spots acquire bluish color.

Record Rf of anethole (dark blue approx. Rf value 0.9 to 0.95) and fenchone (dull blue, approx. Rf value 0.75 to 0.85) in visual light. Reproduce the TLC chart in your record with true colors.

Journal: Page I - 1 & 4; II - 2; III - 3; IV - 6.

CARDAMOM

Elettaria cardamomum   Fam: **Zingiberaceae**

1. Morphology   :   Observe the fruit and note down the external features. Cut the fruit transversely and observe the arrangement of seeds. With the help of a magnifying glass observe the morphological characters of the seed. Refer SCD and draw neat labelled diagrams.

2. TS of Seed   :   Eventhough cardamom is studied under fruit drugs it is the seed which contains more of the active constituents - volatile oils- and hence the study of the seed. Seeds are soaked overnight. Seeds are small and dark brown in color. Observe the raphe carefully and cut sections transverse to the raphe. Take entire sections and observe in CH mount: Calcium oxalate prisms in perisperm tissue. Also observe the arrangement of cells which contain the essential oils. The lignified layer of sclerenchyma can be seen in a stained section. In one another section with water and iodine irrigation, perisperm takes up blue color (Ref. ACD).

3. Powder   :   Observe the color, odor and taste of the freshly powdered seeds. Mount the powder in CH and observe Calcium oxalate crystals -small prisms- in perisperm cells.

Mount little powder in water and irrigate with iodine soln. See the perisperm cells containing starch turning blue. Observe PCD and study and draw the tissues.

4. Extraction of
Cardamom oil :   Take 50 g of cardamom seeds and distil the oil in a steam distillation set. Find out the percentage yield.

Compound	Color	Rf value (Approx.)
α-terpinyl acetate	Dark blue	0.75-0.85
Cineole	Blue	0.65-0.75
Linalool	Grey blue	0.50-0.60
Terpineol	Dark blue	0.40-0.45

5. TLC of Cardamom oil:

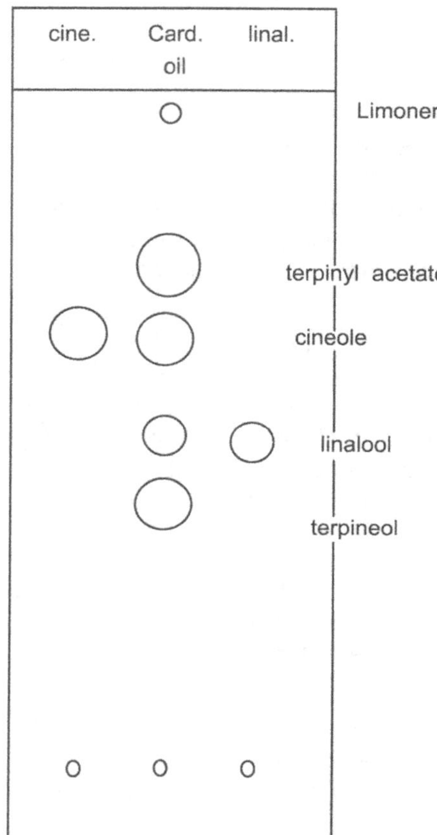

Adsorbent: Silica gel plate.

Solvent System:

Toluene/Benzene: Ethyl acetate (93:7). Take 30 ml (27.9 + 2.1) mixture in a jar. Saturate the chamber for one hour.

Application: All in spot form.

Cardamom oil: 10 µl

(1:10 dilution in Toluene/$CHCl_3$) Cineole: 10 µl (1:30 dilution in $CHCl_3$/Toluene)

Running distance: 10 to 12 cm

Drying:

Air drying for 15-20 min. and then in an oven for 5 min.

Detection:

Cool and spray the plate thoroughly with vanillin - H_2SO_4 reagent and heat at 110 °C for 10 min. under observation. (Do not overheat the plate)

Record Rf value of α-terpinyl acetate, cineole, linalool, terpineol etc. in visual light. Reproduce the TLC chart in your journal.

Journal: Page I - 1; II - 2; III - 3; IV- 4 & 5.

PEPPER

Piper nigrum   Fam: **Piperaceae**

1. Morphology : Observe the entire fruits as well as LS of the fruit with the help of a magnifying lens. Also observe the spike of fruits if available.

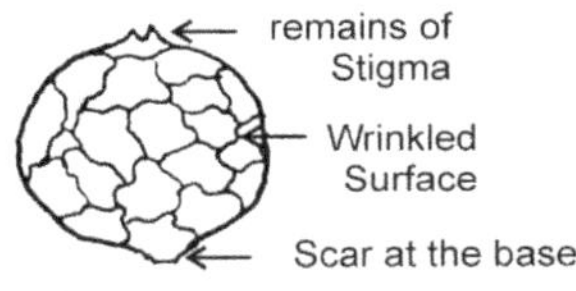

ENTIRE FRUIT XIO

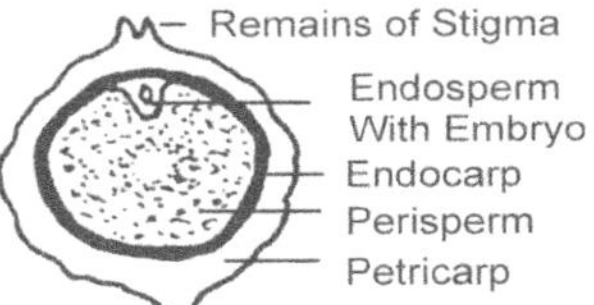

L.S. of Fruit × 10

Fruits are dried berries more or less globular. Surface is dark brown to greyish black and highly reticulated or wrinkled. At the apex the remains of sessile stigmas and at the base a scar indicating the point of attachment to the axis of the spike are seen. Size varies from 3-6 mm. Odor is aromatic and taste pungent.

LS shows a thin pericarp and large perisperm. At the upper portion of the fruit is a minute embryo embedded in small endosperm. Sometimes a cavity is seen in the centre of the perisperm.

2. TS : Fruits are to be soaked overnight in water for taking sections. Observe carefully the longitudinal axis of the fruit (remains of stigma at the top and scar of point of attachment at the base) and cut thin sections at right angles to the axis.

Mount the sections

In CH - observe all tissues as given in ACD (note the differences in the perisperm of cardamom seed and pepper fruit).

In Phloroglucinol + HCl - observe lignified tissues - sclereids below the epidermis and endocarp.

In water preparation irrigated with Iodine perisperm containing starch turning to blue color may be seen (Ref.ACD).

3. Powder : Note the color, odor and taste.

A CH mount shows yellowish color of the slide. A stained powder slide will show lignified sclereids. Water + Iodine - Perisperm turns bluish (PCD).

4. TLC of Pepper extract :

Preparation of the extract:

Take 1 g of Pepper powder and extract by heating under reflux for 15 min. with 10 ml MeOH.

Filter, evaporate the filtrate to 2 ml and use this for TLC studies.

Adsorbent: Silica gel plate.

Solvent System:

Toluene/Benzene: Ethyl acetate (7:3). Take 30 ml (21 + 7) mixture in a jar. Saturate the chamber for one hour.

Application: All in band form. Pepper extract: 20 μl Piperine: 10 μl (dilution 5 mg in 5 ml MeOH)

Running distance: 10 to 12 cm

Drying:

Air drying for 15-20 min. and then in an oven for 5 min.

Detection:

Cool and spray the plate thoroughly with vanillin - H_2SO_4 reagent and heat at 110 $^{\circ}$C for 5-10 min. under observation. When Piperine spots appear lemon yellow, take out the plate (overheating turns yellow spots to violet)

Record Rf value of Piperine (0.5 approx.) in visual light and illustrate the TLC chart in your journal.

Note: TLC of Pepper oil (volatile oil) may also be carried out.

Journal: Page I - 1; II - 2; III - 3; IV - 4.

EPHEDRA

Ephedra species   Fam: **Gnetaceae**

1. Morphology : Observe the young twigs and note the salient macroscopical features as given in SCD. Draw and label the sketches.

2. TS : Stem pieces are to be soaked overnight for taking sections. Present a very thin and an entire section from internodal region. Mount in CH and observe the different tissues as given in ACD. In a stained section observe both lignified tissues (cortical fibres, pericyclic fibres, xylem and pith) and also unlignified fibres present below the ridges. Draw neat labelled diagrams in your record.

3. Powder : Observe color, odor and taste. Observe all the tissues in CH mount. In a stained preparation note both the lignified and unlignified fibres. Illustrate all the sketches as in PCD.

4. TLC : **Preparation of the extract:**

Add 1 g of powdered drug to 10 ml MeOH containing 2 drops of ammonia. Heat on a waterbath for 10 min at 60 °C. Cool, filter and use the filtrate for TLC studies

Adsorbent: Silica gel plate.

Solvent System:

n- butanol: acetic acid : water (4:1:3). Take only 40 ml mixture (20+5+15) in a jar and saturate for 1 to 2 h.

Application: Apply in band form. Along with the extract, reference standard Ephedrine is also to be applied.

Prepared ephedra extract: 20 µl

Ephedrine (1% MeOH soln.): 10 µl

Running distance: 10 cm (takes 2-3 h to develop the plate).

Drying: Air dried for 15-20 min. and in an oven for 10 min.

Detection: Cool, spray with Ninhydrin reagent (saturated soln. of Ninhydrin in ethanol or acetone) and heat in an oven at 110 °C for 5-10 min. under observation till ephedrine appears as reddish colored spot (over heating turns the entire plate reddish)

Record Rf value of Ephedrine (approx. 0.6 - 0.7) in visual light and reproduce the TLC chart in your journal.

Journal: Page I - 1; II - 2; III - 3; IV - 4.

CANNABIS

Cannabis sativa   Fam: **Cannabinaceae**

1. Morphology   :   Observe a fresh specimen/herbarium specimen and study the macroscopical characters as given in SCD. Also illustrate in your record the sketches as given in SCD.

2. Powder   :   Note the color, odor and taste. Mount the powder both in CH and also Phloroglucinol + HCl and study all the tissues appearing from different plant parts as indicated in PCD. Transfer neat labelled diagrams from PCD into your journal.

Journal: Page I - 1; II - 2.

STARCHES

Starches of Rice, Wheat, Maize, Arrow root, Potato and Ginger are usually studied.

Preparation of the starch slide:

1. Take a very small quantity of starch powder on a glass slide and add 2 drops of water and put the coverslip. Add a drop of dil.Iodine soln. at the edge of coverslip and hold a blotting paper on the opposite side. As the water drains the starch grains take up blue color in different gradations.

2. Take little quantity of starch on a glass slide, add 2-3 drops of lactophenol, put a coverglass and observe under LP objective first and then under HP objective to see the hilum, striations etc. clearly. This preparation does not dry up soon and starch grains will not swell up, unlike the starch preparation in water.

Observe the following points for each starch powder both under LP and HP objectives:

1. Simple or Compound
2. Shape
3. Size
4. Hilum - seen or not seen, eccentric or concentric type of hilum, dot like, triradiate, cleft like etc.
5. Striations.

It may be difficult sometimes to differentiate Maize and Arrow root starches. Mount both the starches one under each microscope, observe and remember to identify. Illustrate neat diagrams as per PCD.

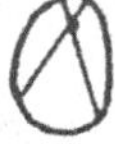  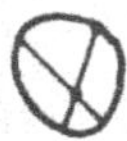

Starch grains under Polarized light: Observe the starch grains of Potato mounted under polarized light and note down the MALTASE cross.

UNORGANIZED DRUGS

Unorganized drugs are studied under the following heads:

(a) Morphology/Macroscopy/Nature as seen in the market sample (SCD)

(b) Identification tests (SCD) - Physical tests

                    Chemical tests and microscopic

                    Characters where possible.

(c) TLC studies wherever possible.

(a) **Morphology:** Shape, size, color, odor, taste etc (SCD).

(b) **Identification tests:** The quality and genuinity can be confirmed by performing certain specific chemical tests. Most of these tests help in distinguishing the authentic drug from the adulterant. These unorganized drugs are supplied to you in powdered form to help you carry out these specific tests.

    (a) **Physical tests:**

        Nature of the powder: Coarse, fine, crystalline, amorphous etc.

        Color of the powder.

        Odor and taste of the powder, if any

        Solubililty of the powdered drug in cold water, warm/hot water, alcohol etc.: Soluble, insoluble, partially soluble, swells up etc.

        Litmus tests: acidic, alkaline, neutral etc.

    (b) **Chemical tests:**

        (SCD) Record your performance in a tabulated form as below:

S. No.	Experiment	Observation	Inference (wherever possible)

After performing the positive tests to confirm the unorganized drug, the negative tests are also to be performed and recorded. (in the examination as well)

Microscopy: Powdered unorganized drugs also reveal important characters in some cases like Aloes. when observed under microscope (PCD).

Source, morphology, active constituents and uses are to be written on the ruled page and the physical tests and chemical tests are to be written on the blank page.

ACACIA

Acacia senegai/A. arabica   Fam: **Leguminosae**

Ruled page   : Source, characters of Acacia tears, active constituents and uses.

Blank page   : Acacia powder

(i)   Physical tests:

- (a)   Nature of powder
- (b)   Color, odor and taste
- (c)   Solubility in water
- (d)   Solubility in alcohol
- (e)   Reaction to litmus (Strong solution of Acacia turns blue litmus red).

(ii)   Chemical tests:

S. No.	Experiment	Observation	Inference
1.	To 5 ml of 10% soln. add 1 ml of clear solution of lead subacetate.	thick white ppt. obtained	(distinction from agar)
2.	**Test for reducing sugars:** A strong solution of acacia is to be boiled thoroughly with dil. HCl directly over the flame in a test tube for 10-15 min. (when hydrolysis is incomplete proper results are not seen). Divide this soln. into two portions. (a) Neutralize the first portion with required volume of NaOH and add equal vol.of Fehling's soln. A & B (2 ml each) and heat again. (b) BaCl$_2$ test : To other hydrolyzed portion add few drops of clear BaCl$_2$ soln.	a brick red ppt. is obtained (ppt. turns yellowish or brownish depending on the proportion of Fehling's solution and neutralization) thick white ppt is not obtained.	Reducing sugars Present (distinction from agar)
3.	To an aq. soln. of acacia add few drops of Iodine solution.	No blue color No brown color	Starch absent Dextrin absent (distinction from agar)
4.	**Test for Tannins:** Add a few drops of FeCl$_3$ to 5 ml of aq.soln. of acacia	No bluish black or green color	Tannins absent

5.	**Test for oxidase** (not performed in the lab) **Tests to distinguish Acacia from Agar :**		
	Solubility (gel formation); Mucilage test (pink coloration);	KOH (canary yellow color) Iodine test (deep crimson to brown color).	

AGAR

Source, morphology of Agar strips, constituents (in brief) and uses to be written on the ruled page of the record.

The following to be written on the blank page:

Agar Powder   :

Physical tests   :   Nature, Color, Odor, Taste

Solubility   :   In cold water swells up

In hot water...

In alcohol...

Litmus test   :

Chemical tests :

S. No.	Experiment	Observation	Inference
1.	**Ruthenium red test:** refer SCD	Powder particles take up pink color	Mucilage present (distinction from Acacia and Tragacanth)
2.	**Reducing sugar test:** Refer SCD, perform the test and write accordingly.	Brick red ppt. of cuprous oxide is formed.	Reducing sugars present.
3.	**Sulphate test:**	Depending upon the hydrolysis, light turbidity to a fairly thick ppt. is obtained	Due to the sulphate ions liberated during hydrolysis (distinction from Acacia, Sterculia and Tragacanth).
4.	Warm a small amount of powder with KOH (do not boil, if boiled it turns to brown)	Canaray yellow color is seen	Distinction from Acacia and Sterculia (Tragacanth also gives canaray yellow color).
5.	**Iodine test :** Add only 1 or 2 drops of iodine solution to dry powder of Agar.	Particles take up crimson to brown color.	Distinction from Acacia and Sterculia
6.	Add aq. Soln. of tannic acid to 2% soln. of Agar (negative test)	No buff colored ppt.	Proteins absent (distinction from Gelatin).
7.	Incinerate Agar in a furnace till ash is formed. Observe the ash under a microscope on glass slide.	Skeletons and spongy spicules of diatoms are seen.	

(this test need not be performed individually, instead in groups)

ALOES

Aloe species   Fam: **Liliaceae**

Source, general morphology of aloes (pieces), active constituents and uses are to be written on the ruled page of the record. on the unruled page the following to be written.

Aloes powder:

(a) **Physical Tests** - Nature, color, odor and taste, Solubility in cold water and alcohol, Litmus test

(b) **Chemical Tests** - To perform the chemical tests, you have to prepare the test solution.

Preparation of test solution: Boil 1 g. of aloes powder with 100 ml water. Cool and add 1g.of kieselguhr, filter and filtrate is used for the following tests. (100 ml test solution is to be shared by 5 or 6 students)

S. No.	Experiment	Observation	Inference
1.	**Borax test for anthranol:** 5 ml of test solution is taken, a pinch of borax is added and heated.	Green colored fluorescence seen (it can be clearly seen when few ml of hot solution is added to a beaker containing water).	Due to aloe emodin anthranol.
2.	**Bromine test:** 2 ml of freshly prepared brominesolution is added to 2 ml test solution.	Heavy yellow ppt. is seen	Due to the formation of tetrabromaloin.

The following tests (3,4 and 5) are performed to differentiate the different varieties and are based on the presence or absence of isobarbaloin. However it is difficult to get the specific colors (results) due to color nuances. Therefore these tests are performed with great care.

S. No.	Experiment	Observation	Inference
3.	**Nitrous acid test:** To 5 ml of test solution add equal volume of Sodium nitrite solution and a few drops of dilute acetic acid.	Pink or purplish color. No color change	Due to isobarbaloin (only curacao and cape aloes). Due to the absence of isobarbaloin (Socotrine arid Zanzibar aloes)

S. No.	Experiment	Observation	Inference
4.	**Nitric acid test:** Add 2 ml of conc.HNO_3 to 5ml of test solution	A brown color changes immediately to green. A deep brownish red color A pale brownish yellow color. Yellowish brown color	cape aloes + Curacao aloes Socotrine aloes Zanzibar aloes
5.	**Klunge's isobarbaloin test/Cupraloin test:** Dilute the test solution with equal volume of water and add a few drops of saturated $CuSO_4$ solution + 1 g. of NaCl + 10 ml alcohol (90%).	Wine red color changes soon to yellow. Feeble wine red color soon changes to yellow. No color change	Curacao aloes Cape aloes Isobarbaloin absent (Zanz. & Socotrine).
6.	**Modified Borntrager's test or Modified anthraquinone test:** To 0.1 g. of the drug add 5ml of 5% $FeCl_3$ solution, 5ml of dil. HCl and boil it on the flame for 10min. Cool the mixture, add 3 ml of benzene. Shake gently and separate the upper benzene layer by decanting or using a separating funnel (this layer must be yellow in color to get proper results). Add 1ml dil. ammonia and shake well.	A cherry pink color appears in the lower ammonical layer	Anthracene derivatives

Microscopy of the powder: Mount the powder in lactophenol and observe the different types of aloes with the aid of PCD.

Note: Students often confuse aloes powder for black catechu or vice versa. By mere organoleptic tests. one can easily distinguish one from other. Do not forget to try this.

TLC of Aloes   :

Preparation of the drug extract.

Take 0.5 g. of powdered aloes and warm with 5 ml MeOH on a water bath for 5 min. Filter and use the clear filtrate for TLC.

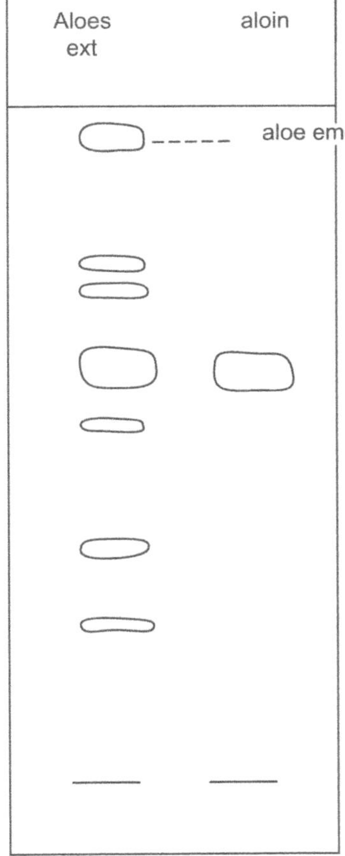

Adsorbent: Silica gel plate

Solvent System:

Ethyl acetate: MeOH: H_2O (100: 13. 5: 10). Take only (30 + 4 + 3).

Application:

Aloes extract: 30 µl Aloin (0.1% in MeOH): 20 µl (both in band form)

Running distance: 10 - 12 cm.

Drying: After the run air dry the plate for 15 min. and then in oven for 10 min.

Detection: Cool and spray the plate thoroughly with 5% ethanolic KOH solution and heat in the oven at 100 °C for 10 min. under observation.

Observe the plate under UV 365 nm. and mark the alcin spots.

Record: Rf values of aloin (yellowish spot). Approximate Rf value: 0.6

Reproduce the results with proper colors in your journal immediately.

Journal: Page I - 1; II - 2; III - 3.

ASAFOETIDA

Ferula foetida   Fam: **Umbelliferae**

As usual Source, morphology, active constituents and uses on the ruled page and on the unruled page the following:

(a) Physical Tests: Form, color, odor, taste, solubility in – cold water, hot water, alcohol and finally litmus test.

(b) Chemical Tests:

S. No.	Experiment	Observation	Inference
1.	a) Solubility in water b) Solubility in alcohol	An emulsion is formed. Partially soluble	
2.	Triturate a little asafoetida with water in a mortar.	Yellowish orange emulsion is formed	
3.	Take a piece of freshly cut surface of asafoetida in a china dish or watch glass. Add 1 or 2 drops of conc. H_2SO_4. Wash the piece in water	Red or reddish brown color is obtained Color changes to violet.	
4.	Take a piece of freshly cut surface of asafoetida in a watch glass/ China dish and add a few drops of 50% HNO_3.	The fractured surface turns greenish in color.	
5.	**Umbelliferone test:** Boil 0.5 g of the drug with 5 ml of 90% alcohol for 2 min., cool and filter. Add 0.5 ml of 10% ammonia solution.	No blue fluorescence	Free Umbelliferone absent.
6.	**Combined Unbelliferone test:** Boil 0.5 g of the drug with 3 ml of conc. HCl and 3 ml of water for 5-10 min., filter and add to the filtrate an equal volume of alcohol and a strong solution of ammonia in excess.	A blue fluorescence is produced.	Due to combined Umbelliferone.

Note: With some market samples of asafoetida, tests 3 and 4 are not answered properly.

BENZOIN

Styrax benzoin   Fam: **Styraceae**

S. tonkinensis

Source, morphology, active constituents and uses of both Sumatra and Siam Benzoin on the ruled page.

Physical and chemical tests on the unruled page.

Benzoin Powder:

Physical Tests: Color, odor, taste, solubility in - cold water, hot water and alcohol. Litmus test.

Chemical Tests:

S. No.	Experiment	Observation	Inference
1.	Heat a small amount of benzoin powder in a dry test tube	Evolves white fumes.	Fumes are of Cinnamic and Benzoic acid
	Condense these fumes on a slide, by holding a slide to the mouth of the test tube.	Crystalline sublimate is seen on the slide.	
2.	Dissolve a small amount of Benzoin in alcohol, either filter of decant the clear upper soln. in another test tube. Add a few drops of alcoholic $FeCl_3$ solution.	No green color	Sumatra benzoin (Siam benzoin gives green color).
3.	Boil 1 g of coarse benzoin powder with 5 ml of 1% $KMnO_4$ soln.	Bitter almond odor	Due to oxidation of Cinnamic acid. (Sumatra benzoin)
		No bitter almond odor.	It is to be presumed that Cinnamic acid is either absent or only in traces. (Siam bezoin)

CATECHU/BLACK CATECHU

Acacia catechu/A. chundra   Fam: **Leguminosae**

Source, morphology, active constituents and uses on the ruled page. Physical and Chemical tests and the microscopy to be done on the unruled page.

Black catechu Powder:

Physical tests : Color, odor, taste, solubility in – cold water, hot water, alcohol and litmus test.

Chemical tests :

S. No.	Experiment	Observation	Inference
1.	To5 ml of 10% filtered aq. soln. of the drug add a few drops of 5% FeCl$_3$ solution Make it alkaline by adding a few drops of NaOH solution.	Dark green color is formed. Green color changes to purple.	Tannins are present. (due to Catechu-Tannic acid)
2.	Add 5 ml of lime water to 2 ml of fresh aq. extract of the drug. Keep the solution for some-time.	Brown color is produced. Gives red ppt.	
3.	Take a small quantity of dry powder on a watch glass or in china dish and add vanillin-HCl (conc.) reagent.	Pink or red color is formed.	Due to the production of phloroglucinol
4.	Prepare an extract of the drug and dip a match stick into it. After drying the stick, dip it into conc. HCl and warm near a flame.	The match stick turns to red or purple-pink.	Due to the reaction of HCl on Catechins Phlo-roglucinol is produced which gives red color with the lignin present in the match stick-wood.
5.	Gambir Fluorescin test: (see pale catechu)	No green fluorescence	(Distinction from pale catechu).

Note: As said under Aloes, one has to make sure that the drug on hand is black catechu based on the organoleptic tests. However, under negative test one can always think of Borntrager's test or for that matter of modified Borntrager's test to confirm.

Microscopy   : Mount a pinch of powder in lactophenol on a glass slide and observe acicular crystals of catechins under a microscope.

CATECHU/PALE CATECHU

Uncaria gambier   Fam: **Rubiaceae**

Source, morphology, active constituents and uses on the ruled page of the record. On the unruled page the following:

Pale Catechu Powder:

Physical Tests   :   Form, color, odor, taste, solubility and litmus test etc.

Chemical Tests   :

S. No.	Experiment	Observation	Inference
1.	Test for tannins:	Same as	
2.	Lime water test:	Black catechu	
3.	Vanillin HCl	(Refer Black	
4.	Match stick test:	catechu)	
5.	Warm 0.5 g of powdered catechu with 2 ml of alcohol, filter and to the filtrate, add 2 ml of NaOH and 2 ml of light petroleum. Shake and allow it to stand. Two layers separate out.	Petroleum layer emits a green fluorescence	This is due to Gambir fluorescin (distinction from black catechu).
6.	Take 2 g of powder, shake well with 5 ml chloroform. Filter after 30 min.	Slight green. color is seen in the filtrate	Due to the presence of Chlorophyll from the leaves of the plant (distinction from black catechu).

To confirm that the given powder is not that of Aloes, one can here as well perform Modified Borntrager's test which should be negative.

Microscopy   :   Refer Black catechu

Note: As there is only one important positive test namely Gambir fluorescin test to distinguish pale catechu form black catechu, this said test has to be performed with all care.

COLOPHONY

Pinus species   Fam: **Pinaceae**

Source, morphology, active constituents and uses on the ruled page.

On the unruled page the following:

Colophony Powder:

Physical Tests   :   Form, color, odor (characteristic when it is freshly powdered), taste, solubility* and litmus tests.

Chemical Tests   :

S. No.	Experiment	Observation	Inference
*	Solubility : In cold water In hot water In alcohol	Insoluble Insoluble Soluble	Distinction from Gelatin (although there is no relationship between the two but students do mistake one for the other based on the color).
1.	Dissolve 0.1 g of powder in 2-3 ml acetic anhydride in a test tube. Add 1 or 2 drops of conc. H_2SO_4 from the sides of the tube (use a dry test tube. Do not add H_2SO_4 directly into the soln. Perform this test carefully.	Purple to violet color is seen.	Due to abietic acid
2.	Dissolve a little fresh powder in 3 ml of light petroleum and filter. To the filtrate add 2-3 times of its volume Copper acetate soln. shake the mixture well.	Emerald green color in the upper petroleum layer.	Due to abietic acid
	(freshly powdered Colophony will answer this test better)		
	Negative test: Prepare about 5 ml test solution, add Picric acid.	No yellow ppt.	Distinction from Gelatin.

GELATIN

Source, nature, constituents and uses on the ruled page. The other details regarding the tests on the unruled page.

Gelatin powder :

Physical Tests : Form, color, odor, taste, solubility and litmus test etc.

Chemical Tests : Gelatin answers the following positive tests due to Proteins

S. No.	Experiment	Observation	Inference
1.	Gelatin powder is heated with soda-lime powder in a dry test tube. **Preparation of the test solution :** Dissolve 0.5 g of gelatin powder in 100 ml water (by heating) and use this for the following tests:	Ammonia is evolved	(Distinction from agar).
2.	Take 5 ml test soln. and add a few drops of Millon's reagent. Heat the white ppt.	A white ppt. is obtained. It turns red.	
3.	To 1 ml of the test Soln. add 1 ml of 10% Mercuric sulphate in 10% H_2SO_4. Boil for 30 sec. Add 2 drops of 1% Sod. nitrite soln.	Red ppt. or red color is obtained.	
4.	Biuret Test : To 3 ml of test soln. add 1 ml of 5% NaOH soln. to make it strongly alkaline. Add 2 drops of 1% $CuSO_4$ soln.	A violet or pink color is formed	
5.	To 3 ml of test soln. add few drops of 10% tannic acid. Heat the test tube again.	White to whitish buff colored ppt. is formed. The ppt. does not dissolve.	(Distinction from agar).
6.	To 3 ml of test soln. add few drops of picric acid.	Yellow ppt. is formed	(Distinction from agar).
7.	Reducing sugar test	No red ppt.	(Distinction from agar).

HONEY

Source, constituents and uses on the ruled page.

The other details as usual on the unruled page.

Physical Tests : Nature, color, odor, taste, solubility (in – cold water, hot water, alcohol) and litmus test.

Chemical Tests :

S. No.	Experiment	Observation	Inference
1.	**Test for reducing sugars :** Dissolve 0.5 ml of honey in 10 ml of water, add 2 ml each of Fehling's soln. A & B and boil.	Red ppt. of copper oxide is seen	Reducing sugars present.
2.	**Selivanoff's test:** Add a crystal of resorcinol to a soln. of honey in water. To this mixture add equal vol. of con.HCl. Warm the test tube on a water bath.	A rose color is obtained.	Due to ketoses like fructose etc.
3.	Mix thoroughly 1 ml of honey with 4 ml of alcohol.	Slight turbidity. More than slight turbidity.	Pure honey Presence of dextrin from added sugars.
4.	**Fiehe's Test:** Shake 10 ml of honey thoroughly with 5 ml of ether till both are miscible. On standing the layers separate. Separate and evaporate the upper ethereal layer in a clean dry porcelain dish. On complete evaporation to dryness, one drop of 1% resorcinol HCl is added.	A transient red coloration is formed. Red coloration persists for sometime.	Natural honey Due to added artificial invert sugars.

Mount a drop of Honey on a glass slide with coverslip and observe under the microscope the different types of pollen grains. These however, are not the ingredients of honey but they do indicate the source of flowers from which the honey bees must have sucked the nectar.

INDIAN TRAGACANTH/ STERCULIA/ KARAYA GUM

Sterculia urens   Fam: **Sterculiaceae**

Genuine tragacanth is not easily available in the Indian markets. what is largely sold in the market under the name 'Tragacanth' is the so called Indian Tragacanth. Hence this is given for practical classes. However, a student should find out the important differences between these two from SCD before proceeding with the actual experiment. As usual, source, morphology, active constituents and uses on the ruled page. On the unruled page the following:

Sterculia Powder:

Physical Tests   :   Form, color, odor (is an important character to distinguish from tragacanth, agar and acacia), taste, solubility (in - cold water, hot water and alcohol) and litmus test.

Chemical Tests   :

S. No.	Experiment	Observation	Inference
1.	**Mucilage test :** Mount a pinch of powder on a slide in Ruthenium red soln. and observe under a microscope.	Particles take pink color	Mucilage present. (Distinction from tragacanth and acacia).
2.	**Reducing sugar test:** Boil 3 ml of sterculia soln. with 1 ml of conc. HCl for 10 min. Divide the soln. in to two parts. Neutralize one portion with NaOH soln. and add 2 ml each of Fehling's soln. A & B and heat again.	Red ppt. is obtained (as it is not easily hydro-lyzable, it is difficult to get dark red ppt.)	Reducing sugars present.
3.	To the other hydrolyzed portion add 1 ml of $BaCl_2$ solution.	No white ppt. or turbidity is obtained.	(Distinction from agar).
4.	Warm little powder with 3 ml KOH soln.	Slight brownish color is formed.	(Distinction from Tragacanth and Agar. Both these give canary yellow color).
5.	Few drops of Iodine soln. is added to a dry sample of Sterculia powder in a test tube or take a little powder on a glass slide and add 1 or 2 drops of Iodine soln., observe under microscope by putting a cover slip.	No blue color in the test tube or under the micro-scope.	Starch absent. Distinction from tragacanth (few starch grains are present) and agar (gives crimson to brown color).

QUANTITATIVE MICROSCOPY
LINEAR/MICROSCOPIC MEASUREMENTS

Microscopic measurements of some tissues, cells, cell contents or plant organs provide valuable information in identifying the drugs or differentiating certain allied drugs or adulterants.

Requirements:

A. Stage Micrometer/Object Micrometer.

B. Eye piece Micrometer/Occular micrometer.

A. Stage micrometer:

It consists of a microscopic slide, on the centre of which is engraved a scale and is fixed by a cover glass. This is to be placed on the stage of microscope, focussed and observed like any other object through the eye piece. Two types of stage micrometers are available:

1. Stage micrometer is of 1 cm length: the scale of which is divided into 10 broad divisions (1 mm each numbered as 0, 10, 20, ... 100) and each broad division (0 to 10) is further divided into 10 more finer divisions (0.1 mm each). Thus there are 100 divisions in the scale and each smallest division is said to be 0.1 mm or 100 μm.

2. Here the stage micrometer is of 1 mm length and this scale also is divided in the same way as mentioned above. But each broad division here is 0.1 mm (l00 μm) and smallest division is 0.01 mm or 10 μm (microns). The mm scale being more accurate, the same is recommended for any accurate measurements.

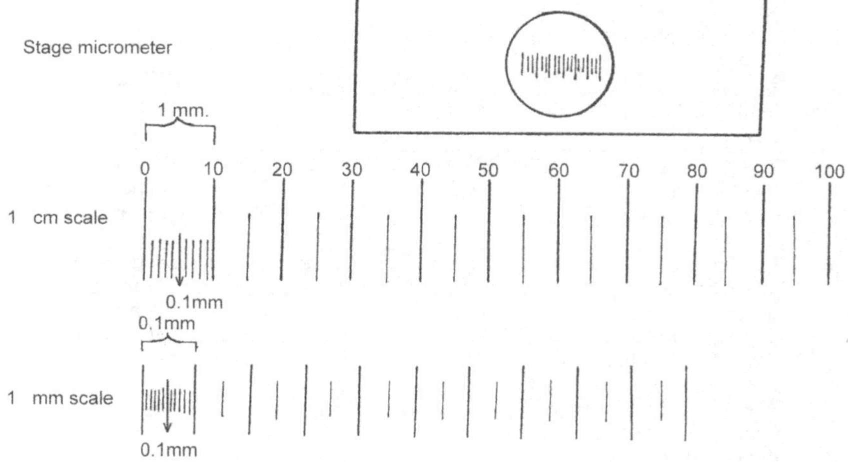

B. Eye piece micrometer

Different types of eye piece micrometers are available. It consists of a glass disc with a scale on it and is fixed or kept inside the eye piece. It may be an ordinary eye piece in which the scale is fixed or an eye piece which is adjustable on the upper portion, or the eye piece (with the scale) fixed to a box having a knob to move the scale to its left or right.

This scale is also normally divided into 100 divisions and may or may not be numbered.

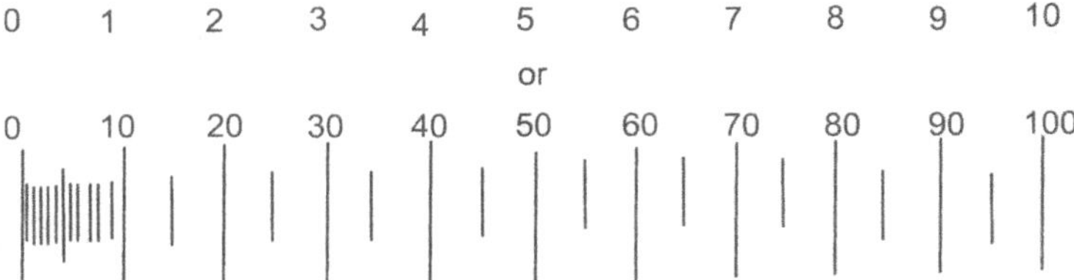

STANDARDIZATION OR CALIBRATION OF THE EYE PIECE MICROMETER

The scale of the eye piece micrometer (graticule) is an arbitrary scale and this has to be standardized before we use it for any measurement. Standardization of eye piece micrometer can be made using either a low power objective or a high power objective. Needless to mention, the value varies if standardization is done with LPO and measurement is done on HPO. Focus the stage micrometer under LPO using 10X eye piece. Replace the eye piece with an eye piece micrometer. Now both the scales are seen in the field of view. Adjust the scales in such a way that both the scales are superimposed.

Carefully adjust and see that 1st divisions of both scales (on the left side) coincide with each other. Then find out which other division of both the scales (on the right side) coincide. For example 100 divisions of Eye Piece Micrometer (EPM) coincide with ..... divisions of SM (stage micrometer) or 100 divisions of SM coincide with.... divisions of EPM. If it is not possible to see 100 divisions, take anywhere from the middle 50 divisions or so. Sometimes it may be difficult to adjust zeros of both scales as they are seen at the extreme left edge. It is advisable to take more than 10 divisions of any scale. More number of divisions will give more accurate results/values.

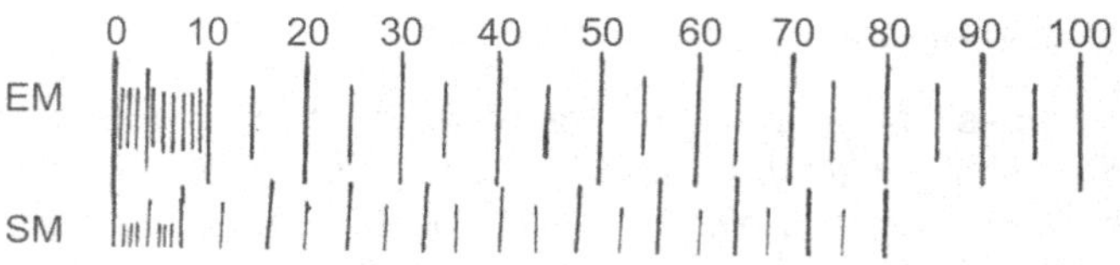

80 div. of EPM coincide with 100 div. of SM (mm scale)

Calculate the value of each EPM division as follows:

(a) SM is of 1 mm length and is divided into 100 div.

Each div. of SM is = 1 mm/100 = 1000 μm /100 = 10 μm and then, 80 div. of EPM coincide with 100 div. of SM.

Therefore 80 div. of EPM = 100 x 10 μ = 1000 μm

1 div. of EPM = 1000 μm/80 = 12.5 μm.

(b) SM used is of 1 cm length and is divided into 100 div. Each division of stage micrometer is = 1 cm/100 = 0.1 mm.

i.e., 10000 μm/100 = μm

If 100 divisions of EPM coincide with 8 div. of SM, 1 div. of EPM coincide with 8 x 100 μm/100 = 8 μm.

Students are advised not to get confused with EPM & SM div.

Tissues/particles that are usually given for measurements:

Length of fibres of Cinchona, Cassia, Trichomes of Senna, Tea etc.; Starch grains (Potato), acicular raphides (squill), Length and breadth of oil glands of clove as seen in TS, diameter of xylem vessels of Quassia as seen in TS, diameter of pollen grains of any flowers etc, Students must aquaint themselves with all the above items. Any one of the items may be asked in the examination.

Precautions to be taken:

Mount starch grains in lactophenol/water. Learn the technique of isolation and mounting of pollen grains from flowers. While measuring lignified tissues like Quassia vessels, tea trichomes etc. it is better to stain them before measuring. Take care not to measure broken pieces. TS of Clove and powder of Squill may be mounted in CH.

Actual measurement of the given object:

Make one or two preparations of the given object for measurement (TS/powder/pollen grains). Replace the SM by the slide. The EPM can be moved in any direction by rotating the same. Find out the number of divisions the object has covered. Say 8. This has to be multiplied with your standard value/reference value. Take 10 such readings. While measuring fibres, trichomes, starch grains, take readings of various sizes - small, average and big. Record your observations as follows and calculate as given below:

Length of fibres of Cinchona

S. No.	Number of divisions covered by the EPM	Actual length of Fibres (No. of divisions of EPM × Std. value of each EPM)
1.	45	45 × 8 = 360 μm.
2.	100	100 × 8 = 800 μm.
to	.....	
10.	.....	

Take the average of 10 readings (.....μ)

Result and Report: The length of Cinchona fibres varies from minimum to average to maximum :

360 μm to ..... μm. to 1440 μm.

VEIN-ISLET NUMBER &
VIENLET TERMINATION NUMBER

Vein-islet: Is a term used to indicate the minute areas of photosynthetic tissues encircled by the ultimate divisions of the vascular strands.

Vein-islet Number: The number of vein-islets per square mm is termed as the VIN.

Veinlet Termination Number: An ultimate free end or termination of a veinlet is called as veinlet termination and the number of such veinlet terminations/ square mm is termed as VTN.

Preparation and Mounting of the Material:

1. Cut 3-4 pieces of the leaf (fresh or dried) from the middle portion of the lamina avoiding midrib and margin. The size of each piece must be smaller than that of the coverslip.

2. Take these in a test tube and boil in strong chloral hydrate soln. directly over the flame or in a waterbath, till they are cleared properly.

3. In case of thick leaves which are difficult to clear with CH soln. treat them first with chlorinated soda soln. for bleaching and with 10% HCl to dissolve the calcium oxalate crystals and finally boil in strong CH soln.

4. Transfer these leaf pieces to a watch glass, pick up a piece using a brush and mount on the slide in CH soln. with lower surface facing upwards so that the veins which are more prominent on the lower surface are seen clearly under the microscope.

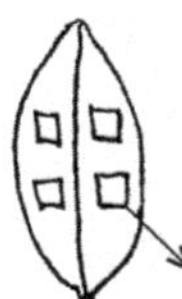

Method

1. To carry out this experiment, use 5x or 6x eye piece and LP objective.

2. Focus stage micrometer (1 mm) and fix the **Camera Lucida** (Camera Lucida is an instrument having a pair of prisms which help in exact reproduction of microscopical image on a drawing paper). To fix the camera lucida remove the eye piece, insert the ring of the camera lucida into the draw tube of the microscope, replace the eyepiece and see that the upper part of the camera lucida rests on the eyepiece in such a way that the aperture of the camera lucida is in line with that of eye piece. Tighten the screw of the camera lucida to the draw tube.

3. Place a drawing sheet (preferably black sheet) on the working table, on the same side of the microscope where camera lucida is fixed (in other words, if camera lucida is fixed on the right side, paper also is to be placed on the right side).

4. The aperture of the camera lucida is partially covered by the portion of the prism. While observing through the camera lucida, adjust your eye in such a way that you are able to see the micrometer scale through the eye piece as well as the prism portion. That is how the image looks superimposed and can be traced on the drawing sheet.

5. Using a white/yellow pencil mark the first and last line of the stage micrometer (mm scale). Measure these two points, join them and make a square (I mm ^{2}).

6. Remove the stage micrometer and mount the slide with the leaf specimen and focus the same now. Adjust the square drawn on the paper in such a way that it lies exactly in the middle of the field of vision. Close the iris diaphragm partially and adjust the illumination.

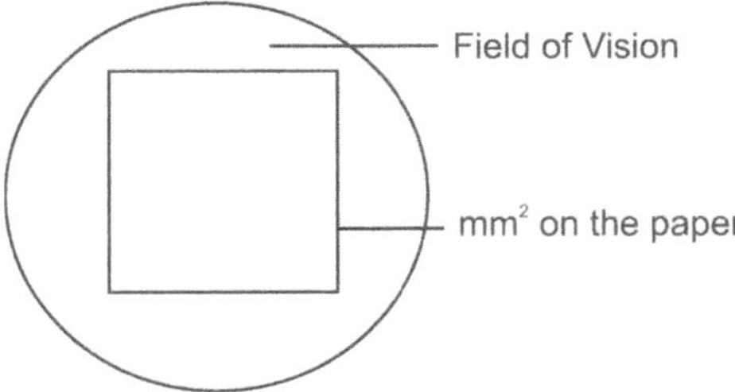

7. Now the image of the leaf piece mounted appears to overlap (superimpose) the square on the drawing sheet.

8. Start from any one side and trace all the vein islets inside the square and also complete those which are on the boundary of square. Along with vein-islets trace the veinlet terminations also which are inside the square only.

9. Draw thick and thin veins as you see in the specimen to show some naturality. Do not move the camera lucida or drawing sheet, once you have begun to trace the veins.

10. At this juncture show your preparation as well as tracing of veins to your concerned teacher before the adjustments get disturbed.

11. Thus to get exact and standard values, it is necessary to take readings from 4 contiguous squares (or rectangle as the case may be) and trace the vein-islets within it. But in actual practice, it is difficult to get the entire rectangle within the field or view. As the students at this stage are only

learning the technique, they may draw one another square of the same size, choose the adjacent area of the specimen and trace the vein-islets and terminations.

Counting and Calculation:

First count all the vein-islets in the square. Count also the ones which are on the border lines of any two adjacent sides (but not from opposite sides) i.e., bottom and left/left and top/top and right/right and bottom. Also count the terminations which are only inside the square. Use different numbers for vein-islets and veinlet terminations (i.e., 1, 2, 3/ I, II, III etc.). Calculate the average values obtained from both the squares.

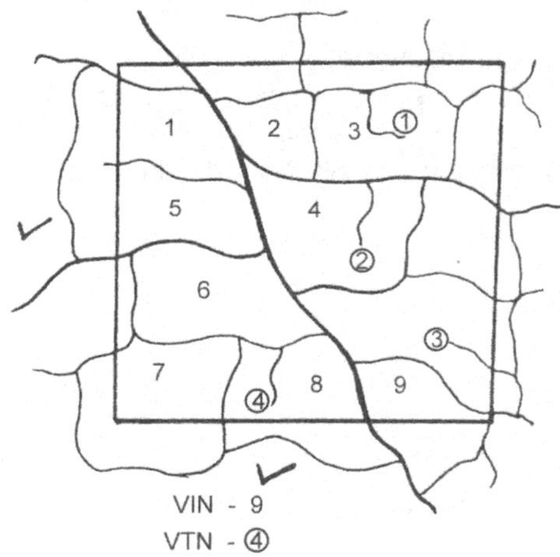

Report/ Result

The vein-islet number of Datura leaf is ....

The veinlet termination number is ....

Attach this sheet to your record (in blank page and write the procedural details on the ruled page).

In the practical examination, you are expected to write the definition, should know the right combination of eyepiece and objective. Get examiner's approval as and when you finish taking the readings.

Suggestion: This experiment has to be completed in 30-45 min. time so that you feel at ease in completing the same in the examination as well with the pressure of time.

STOMATAL INDEX

Definitions:

Stomatal Index : is the percentage proportion of stomata and epidermal cells plus stomata. In other words

$$SI = \frac{S}{E+S} \times 100$$

Where S = No. of stomata per unit area

E = No. of ordinary epidermal

cells in the same unit area.

Stomatal Number : is the number of stomata per square mm of epidermis.

For a given species the stomatal index is highly constant but stomatal number differs according to the age of the leaf.

Preparation of sample:

Leaf sample is to be prepared according to the same procedure that is given for vein islet number, in case of thick leaves where it is not possible to take epidermal peelings. A simple method of preparing the material is by mounting a peeling of the lower epidermis (in case of dorsiventral leaves) or of upper and lower epidermal layer (in case of isobilateral leaves SI is to be determined separately for UE & LE). A peeling can be easily taken by partially cutting one of veins with a blade on the lower epidermal region and pulling it. A thin white membraneous layer comes out along with the vein. Place this on a glass slide cut and remove the thick vein portion attached to it, if any, add few drops of CH soln. and place the coverslip, taking care that no air bubbles creep in. If air bubbles appear just hold the slide over the flame for a short while to remove them and finally place the coverslip. Do not heat or boil this layer in CH, as the epidermal cell walls cannot be seen clearly after boiling. The peeling must be sufficiently big enough, so that it covers the entire field of view when mounted under HP objective.

Method:

1. Use 10 × eye piece and high power objective.

2. For Stomatal number, take 1 mm square with the help of a Stage Micrometer according to the procedure given under VIN.

3. For SI put a circle which is slightly smaller than that of field of view on the tracing paper. Make the edge of the circle more darker/thicker so that it is clearly visible while observing through the camera lucida.

4. Fix the camera lucida to the microscope (see VIN) and looking through it under LP adjust the paper in such a way that the circle/square is clearly visible in the centre of the field of view.

5. Focus the sample under HP objective, adjust for proper illumination and replace the camera lucida and confirm whether you are able to see the sample superimposed on the circle/square or not.

6. For stomatal number one has to mark only the stoma while for SI both stomata as well as epidermal cells are to be marked.

7. Before marking care has to be taken that both stomata and epidermal cells are clearly seen. Mark all the stomata (a stoma includes 2 guard cells and the stomal aperture) on the tracing paper as and then the epidermal cells including the subsidiary cells which surround the stoma as 'X'. While marking the epidermal cells, in case these are in large number, start marking from one corner and complete at the other end. If trichomes of either type-covering or glandular- are seen, the base of each one is to be considered as equivalent to one epidermal cell unit. The stomata and epidermal cells that are lying on the border-line are to be taken into account and so are to be marked provided they are atleast 50% inside the boundary. Repeat the experiment by selecting one another area. As usual at this juncture obtain the concerned teacher's approval of your readings.

8. Counting: In case of stomatal number, count the number of stomata and take the average of 2 or more readings. For stomatal index first count and number the stomata and thereafter the epidermal cells on the black sheet (use different colors to differentiate stomata from epidermal cells).

9. Calculate the values and take the average of atleast 2 readings.

10. Attach the black sheet with the tracings on it to a blank page of the record and write the definition, procedure etc. on the ruled page of the record.

Suggestion: This experiment has to be completed in 30-45 min. time so that you feel at ease in completing the same in the examination as well with the pressure of time.

$$\frac{S}{E+S} \times 100 =$$

$$\frac{5}{20+5} \times 100 = 20$$

PALISADE RATIO

Definition

Palisade Ratio is defined as the average number of palisade cells below each epidermal cell, and is of diagnostic value in differentiating the species. It remains constant within a range for a given plant species. The value does not alter in samples of different localities or according to the age of the plant. However it does differ from species to species and hence important. It has but one limitation like, this cannot be done for monocot leaves as the mesophyll in the monocot is not differentiated. But we do not require large portions of leaf pieces to perform this exercise unlike the other two experiments.

Preparation of the material

1. Take small pieces of leaf from the apex, middle and basal portion of the lamina of young & old leaves. (If possible, peel off the lower epidermis and then cut the pieces).

2. Boil gently and carefully in a test tube 4 to 5 such leaf pieces in about 5 ml strong soln. of CH till the dark green color of leaf turns light green. Avoid over heating otherwise either the epidermal layer gets separated as a thin transparent sheath or the edges of cells will not be visible under the microscope.

3. Pick up one of the pieces carefully and place it on the glass slide with its upper epidermal layer uppermost (one can differentiate the upper surface from lower surface by observing the prominent veins on the lower surface).

4. Add 3-4 drops of CH soln. and put the coverslip carefully.

5. Focus under LP objective first and then under HP objective with l0x or l5x eye piece.

6. Cut down the illumination partially and focus the upper epidermal layer (in case you are mounting lower epidermis you will find large number of stomata. Then remove the coverslip and turn the leaf piece upside down).

7. Try to see 4 clear contiguous epidermal cells and then turndown slowly the fine adjustment knob. The epidermal cells disappear from the vision and instead round, light green, closely packed palisade cells are seen. Note that at one and the same time both epidermal cells and palisade cells cannot be seen.

8. Fix the camera lucida as mentioned in the earlier experiments and arrange the black colored drawing sheet.

9. Before you start drawing make sure that you see both the epidermal and palisade cells very clearly.

10. Trace 4 contiguous epidermal cells using a color pencil. Make these line diagrams darker. Avoid trichomes & stomata.

11. Move the fine adjustment, focus palisade layer and draw the palisade cells inside all the 4 epidermal cells. Also draw those which are on the outer boundary of 4 epidermal cells. At this juncture get your teacher's approval.

12. Change the area of the sample and repeat the experiment.

13. Mark all the palisade cells inside the boundary and those which are 50% or more inside the outer boundary of 4 epidermal cells. Divide the number of palisade cells by 4.

This gives the average number of palisade cells under each epidermal cell.

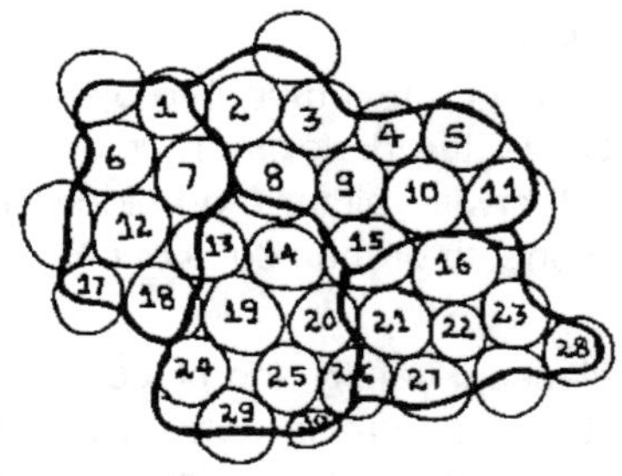

$$PR = \frac{30}{4} = 7.5$$

Attach this sheet in your journal and write the procedural details.

MISCELLANEOUS DRUGS

Some of the drugs given below, as mentioned in the syllabus are to be studied only for their source, active constituents and uses and as such are often kept in the practical examination for identification (spotters).

Pharmacognosy I

Alginate, Brahmi, Vinca, Tulsi, Shankapushpi, Lehsun, kaolin, Guar Gum, Kesar, Myrrh, Asafoetida, Male Fern, Balsam of Tolu, Chrysarobin, Turpentine oil, Storax, Asoka, Arjuna, Wild Cherry bark, Bees wax, Banafsha, Cantharidis and Lycopodium.

Pharmacognosy II

Aswagandha, Curcuma, Punarnava, Rasna, Saussurea, Belladonna root, Jalap, Senega, Satavari, Vaj, Picrorhiza, Ipomoea, Chirata, Kalmegh, Lobelia, Colchicum (corm and seeds), Kapur Kachri, Jatamansi, Gokhru, Lemon peel, Orange peel, Kokum Butter, Kaladana, Bael, Dill, Nutmeg, Myrobalan, Psoralea (Bavchi), Colocynth, Amla, Mustard, Physostigma, Pipal and Vidang.

COMMON REAGENTS USED BY STUDENTS

Anisaldehyde–sulfuric acid:

For spraying TLC plates of Volatile oils. Take 1 ml anisaldehyde in 20ml glacial acetic acid. Mix 170 ml methanol followed by 10 ml conc. sulfuric acid. This reagent is unstable and cannot be kept for a long time. And also should not be used when color changes to reddish violet.

Bromine Water: One of the reagent for testing Aloes. Saturated soln. of bromine (to be prepared in a fuming chamber).

Chloral hydrate soln.: 250 g of chloral hydrate to be dissolved in 100 ml water (common clearing agent). It clarifies cell walls and removes chlorophyll, starch, proteins, mucilage but retains calcium oxalate crystals, fats and oils.

Chloral hydrate (Strong) soln.: Dissolve 400 g of CH in 100 ml water. This soln. is useful in clearing thick tissues, to remove chlorophyll completely which is required in case of Quantitative Microscopic experiments like determination of Vein-islet number and to see clearly the calcium oxalate crystals in the mesophyll of solanaceous drugs.

Chlorinated soda soln.:

(i) Take 250 ml of water and dissolve 150 g of Sodium carbonate.

(ii) Take 100 g of chlorinated lime in a mortar, add 750 ml of water and mix properly.

Mix (1) & (ii), shake occasionally for 4-5 h. and filter.

Use: Used in clearing/bleaching the leaf pieces in Quantitative microscopy experiments.

Corallin Soda soln.:

Solution I: Prepare 5% soln. of corallin in alcohol (90%).

Solution II: Dissolve 25 g Sodium carbonate in 100 ml water. Keep solutions I & II separately. Mix I & II in the proportion 1:20 when required. This mixture is to be used within a week. This is used to stain the mucilage of Squill.

Dragendorff's Reagent:

Solution A: Dissolve 8.5 g bismuth subnitrate and 100 g tartaric acid in 400 ml water.

Solution B: Dissolve 160 g Potassium iodide in 400 ml water. When required mix 5 ml of soln.A and 5 ml soln. B, 100 ml of water and 20 g tartaric acid.

Use: To detect alkaloids (Alkaloids of Kurchi, Aconite, Nux vomica etc. Spraying reagent as well). For TLC of Solanaceous drugs, after spraying the plate with Dragendorff's reagent, the spots appear very dull. In order to intensify the appearance, the plate is to be again sprayed carefully with 5% aqueous sodium nitrite soln.

Fehling's Solutions: To detect reducing sugars of Agar, Acacia, Sterculia, Tragacanth, Honey etc.

Fehling's soln. A: Add 7 g of Copper sulfate and 0.1 ml sulfuric acid to make 100 ml in distilled water.

Fehling's soln. B: Add 35 g of Sodium potassium tartrate and 15.4 g sodium hydroxide to make 100 ml in distilled water.

Mix equal volumes of both soln. when required.

Ferric chloride soln.: 5% soln. of Ferric chloride in water (5 g in 100 ml water). This is used to detect Tannins (Catechu both black and pale).

Ferric chloride soln. (alcoholic): 5% soln. of ferric chloride in alcohol 90% . Used to detect phenols (clove oil, cinnamon oil).

Glycerin soln.: 50% soln. of glycerin in water. Used as temporary mount. Keeps the section and powder from drying for a considerable time.

Iodine Solution: Dissolve 2g of Iodine and 3 g of Potassium iodide in 100 ml water. Used to stain starch preparations. Also used in the chemical tests for Agar, Acacia, Tragacanth and Sterculia and to distinguish Indian Squill from European Squill.

Iodine-Chloroform reagent: 0.5% soln. of Iodine in chloroform. Used for TLC studies of Ipecac.

Iodine-HCl reagent: Alcoholic iodine soln : Dissolve 1 g iodine and 1 g of potassium iodide in 100 ml ethanol.

Alcoholic HCl soln.: Mix 50 ml of 25% HCl with 50 ml of ethanol. Spraying reagents for TLC studies of Coffee and Tea.

Lactophenol: Add 20 g of phenol, 20 g lactic acid, 40 g glycerin to 20 ml distilled water and dissolve.

Use: To observe aloes powder, starch grains etc.

Millon's reagent (Mercuric nitrate soln.): Dissolve 1 ml of mercury in 9 ml fuming nitric acid (Caution? During the reaction keep the mixture cool). Add equal volume of distilled water. Used to detect proteins present in Gelatin for example.

Ninhydrin Reagent: Dissolve 0.3 g ninhydrin in 100 ml n.butanol and add 3 ml acetic acid. Specially used to detect amino acids (we use it to detect ephedrine, an alkaloidal amine).

Phloroglucinol soln.: 1 g of phloroglucinol is dissolved in 100 ml alcohol.

Use: A common staining reagent. Lignified tissues are stained reddish with phloroglucinol & conc. HCl (1: 1).

Phosphomolybdic acid reagent: 20 g of phosphomolybdic acid is dissolved in 100 ml alcohol. This is used to identify a phenolic ether-anethole present in Fennel oil (TLC spraying reagent).

Potassium permanganate-sulfuric acid reagent: This again is used as a spraying reagent to detect a ketone-fenchone-in fennel oil. This reagent is to be prepared carefully. Dissolve 1 g potassium permanganate in 30 ml sulfuric acid (keep the beaker containing H_2SO_4 in a vessel with ice cubes and slowly add pot. permanganate).

Ruthenium Red soln.: Dissolve 0.008 g of Ruthenium red in 10 ml lead acetate soln. (10%). (To be prepared fresh).

Used to stain the mucilage present in drugs like Agar, Sterculia, Isapgol, Linseed.

Vanillin-Hydrochloric acid reagent: 1% soln. of vanillin in conc. HCl. Used to detect catechins (Catechu-black and pale)

Vanillin-Sulfuric acid reagent:

Soln. A: 1% soln. of vanillin in ethanol.

Soln. B: 5% soln. of sulfuric acid in ethanol.

Mix equal volumes of A and B when required. This again is a common reagent to spray essential oils.

HOW TO SCORE HUNDRED PERCENT MARKS IN THE TLC EXERCISE ?

First you have to identify the powdered drug without the help of any book. Having identified, you must say on what basis you have identified? In other words you must give one or two important characters and support these with neat diagrams.

For example: I have identified the given drug as Senna on the basis of the following diagnostic characters:

1. Unicellular, non lignified, warty trichomes ..... diagram.
2. Crystal sheath or crystal fibre ..... diagram.

As we know Senna contains anthracene derivatives. I would like to confirm the drug by carrying out a TLC experiment. For this, may I request you to supply me Senna extract, reference standards like Sennoside A, B, C and D for comparison purposes ?

At this stage show this to examiner and get it approved. This carries one third of the total marks. By chance, you have identified the powder wrong, one more chance may be given by deducting 2 mark from the total of one third. If one is again wrong, the powdered drug will be announced by the examiner and for the rest of the expt., you will be valued only for 50% of the total marks.

Run the plate by following the given instructions. Show the plate to the examiner after spraying etc. This part carries again one third of the total marks. To get the remaining one third, illustrate the TLC plate through a neatly drawn chart in proper colors and with Rf values for the main constituents.

HOW TO PROCEED WITH MICROSCOPIC MEASUREMENTS IN THE EXAMINATION?

MICROSCOPIC MEASUREMENTS

1. **Aim of the experiment:** To measure the length of fibres in the given powdered drug.

2. **Requirements:**

   (a) Microscope   (b) Stage micrometer

   (c) Eye piece micrometer   (d) Material to be measured

3. **Procedure:**

   (i) Standardization of Eye piece micrometer: The Stage micrometer supplied is of 1 cm/ 1 mm size which is divided into 100 divisions. So each division is 100 μm/ 10 μm.

   (ii) 'X' divisions of Eye piece micrometer coincide with 'Y' divisions of Stage micrometer. (Take examiner's signature)

   Since 1 dive of Stage micrometer = 100 μm / 10 μm. 'X' div. of Eye piece micrometer = 'Y' × 100 μm / 10 μm.

   Therefore 1 div. of EPM = $\dfrac{\text{'y' x 100 } \mu m / 10 \, \mu m.}{\text{'x'}}$ = $z \, \mu m..$

(iii)   Measurement of fibres:

S. No.	No. of dive(EPM)	Measurement in microns	Remarks
1.	50	$50 \times z$ μm.	Minimum
to	Take the average value of 10 readings.		
10	(take examiners sign. for one of the readings)		maximum

Result : The length of the fibres in the given powder is

From ..... μm (min .) to..... μm (ave.) to ..... μm (max.)

Model Paper

First Sessional Practical Examination
Pharmacognosy I

Third B. Pharm **Time: 3 hrs.**

Max. Marks: 50

1. Identify the given two drugs and write their common name, botanical source, family, active constituents and uses 6
2. Identify and write the morphology of the given specimen with a labelled sketch 4
3. Identify the given powder and carry out the TLC study for its active principles ..... 3 + 3 + 3 = 9

or

Identify the given unorganized drug by physical and chemical tests. Report all the tests 9

4. Make microscopic preparation of the given sample and present the slide(s) with a neat labelled diagram. Describe the various tissues broadly ..... 4+1+5= 10
5. Analyze the given mixture of three powdered drugs giving reasons 15
6. Viva-voce..... 6

Second Sessional Practical Examination
Pharmacognosy I

Third B. Pharm **Time: 3 hrs.**

Max .Marks: 50

1. Identify the given two drugs and write their common name, botanical source, family, active constituents and uses 6
2. Identify and write the morphology of the given specimen with a labelled sketch 5
3. Make microscopic measurement of .....(take atleast 10 readings) 10
4. Make microscopic preparation of the given sample and present the slide(s) with a neat labelled diagram. Describe the various tissues broadly ..... 4 + 1 + 4 = 10
5. Analyze the given mixture of three powdered drugs giving reasons 18

Third Sessional/University Practical Examination

Third B. Pharm **Pharmacognosy I** **Time: 4 hrs.**

Max. Marks: 60

1. Identify the given two drugs and write their common name, botanical source, family, active constituents and uses 5
2. Identify and write the morphology of the given specimen with a labelled sketch ... 3
3. Identify the given powder and carry out the TLC study for its active principles ..... $3 + 2\frac{1}{2} + 2\frac{1}{2} = 8$

or

Identify the given unorganized drug by physical and chemical tests. Report all the tests... 8

4. Make microscopic measurement of ..... (take atleast 10 readings) 8
5. Make microscopic preparation of the given sample and present the slide(s) with a neat labelled diagram. Describe the various tissues broadly..... 4+1+5= 10
6. Analyze the given mixture of three powdered drugs giving reasons 18
7. Viva-voce 8

First Session Practical Examination

Final B. Pharm **Pharmacognosy II** **Time: 3 hrs.**

Max. Marks: 50

1. Identify the given two drugs and write their common name, botanical source, family, active constituents and uses 6
2. Identify and write the morphology of the given specimen with a labelled sketch 3
3. Make microscopic preparation of the given sample and present the slide(s) with a neat labelled diagram. Describe the various tissues broadly..... 4 + 1 + 5 = 10
4. Define Stomatal index/Vein-islet number/Palisade ratio and determine the value for the given leaf. (take two readings) 9
5. Analyze the given mixture of three powdered drugs giving reasons 15
6. Viva-voce 7

Second Sessional Practical Examination

Final B. Pharm   **Pharmacognosy II**   **Time: 3 hrs.**
                                                          Max. Marks: 50

1. Identify the given two drugs and write their common name, botanical source, family, active constituents and uses 9

2. Identify and write the morphology of the given specimen with a labelled sketch 4

3. Identify the given powder and carry out the TLC study for its active principles....   3 + 3 + 3 = 9

4. Make microscopic preparation of the given sample and present the slide(s) with a neat labelled diagram. Describe the various tissues broadly.... 4 + 1 + 5 = 10

5. Analyze the given mixture of three powdered drugs giving reasons 18

Third Sessional/University Practical Examination

Final B. Pharm   **Pharmacognosy II**   **Time: 4 hrs.**
                                                          Max. Marks: 60

1. Identify the given two drugs and write their common name, botanical source, family, active constituents and uses..... 5

2. Identify and write the morphology of the given specimen with a labelled sketch 3

3. Identify the given powder and carry out the TLC study for its active principles ..... $3 + 2\frac{1}{2} + 2\frac{1}{2} = 8$

4. Make microscopic preparation of the given sample and present the slide(s) with a neat labelled diagram. Describe the various tissues broadly ..... 4 + 1 + 5 = 10

5. Define Stomatal index/Vein-islet number/Palisade ratio and determine the value for the given sample (take two readings)..... 8

6. Analyze the given mixture of three powdered drugs giving reasons 18

7. Viva-voce 8